AF797125

MEDICAL THINGS EXPLAINED

MTE

by Stacie the PA

Menopause 101:

What Every Husband Should Know About the Change

By Stacie the PA

For permission requests, contact:

Stacie the PA
medicalthingsexplained@gmail.com
www.StaciethePA.com

Printed and published in the United States of America.
First Edition – 2025

Disclaimer

This book is for **educational purposes only** and is not intended to replace individualized medical advice, diagnosis, or treatment.
Always seek the guidance of your own qualified healthcare provider with any questions about a medical condition, medication, or treatment plan. Never disregard or delay professional medical advice because of something you have read in this book.

While every effort has been made to ensure the accuracy of the information presented, medicine evolves rapidly, and recommendations may change. Readers are encouraged to verify details with updated professional guidelines or their healthcare provider.

The author and publisher assume no liability for any injury, loss, or damage resulting from the use or misuse of the information contained herein.

Acknowledgments & Dedication

I would like to extend my heartfelt gratitude to the many healthcare professionals I have had the privilege of working with over the past two decades. From teachers and professors who laid the foundation of my medical education to the clinicians and support teams who bring compassion and excellence to patient care every day—you have each contributed to this work in meaningful ways.

To my colleagues in medicine—physicians, physician assistants, nurse practitioners, nurses, anesthetists, pharmacists, therapists, social workers, and medical assistants—thank you for your expertise, mentorship, and shared commitment to helping patients heal and thrive. To the administrative staff, technicians, and countless behind-the-scenes professionals who make quality care possible, your work is deeply valued and never unseen.

Your collaboration, teaching, and dedication have shaped not only my career but also the clarity and empathy that guide these books. Each lesson learned, each patient helped, and each conversation shared has strengthened my belief that education is one of the most powerful tools in healthcare.

This book—and the entire 101 Series—is dedicated to all of you who continue to serve, teach, and lead with heart. Thank you for inspiring me to make medicine more understandable, more compassionate, and more human.

Table of Contents

Introduction

Game On: You're on the Same Team

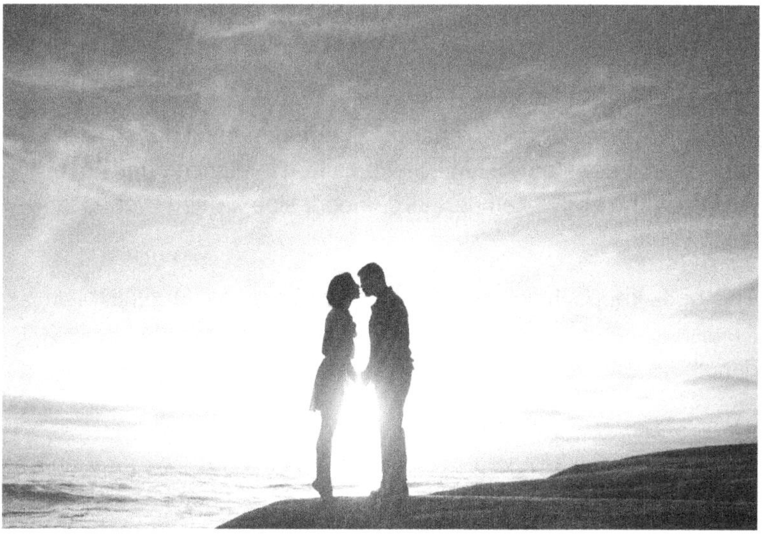

For Partners (Playbook)

Let's start here: menopause is not a disease—it's a transition. It's the second-half of the game that every woman eventually plays, but most men never get the rulebook. Suddenly the person you love may not sleep, may sweat through the sheets, or may cry for no reason—and you're standing there thinking, *What just happened?*

This book gives you the playbook you never got. You'll learn what's actually going on inside her body, what helps (and what doesn't), and how to keep your relationship solid through all of it. You don't need a medical degree—just curiosity, patience, and a willingness to show up.

For Women (Huddle)

Menopause is a normal, natural phase that marks the end of menstrual cycles. It doesn't happen overnight and it doesn't define you. What it *does* do is shift hormones that influence nearly every system in the body—temperature, mood, sleep, heart, bones, and sexual health.

This book keeps things simple. It explains medical terms in plain English, gives you evidence-based options, and includes tools you can share with your partner so you don't have to navigate this alone.

How to Use This Book

- Each chapter begins with a **clinical title** so you can quickly find what you need.
- Beneath that title, a **sports-style subheading** connects the science to real-life teamwork.
- Within the chapter, you'll find **For Partners (Playbook)** and **For Women (Huddle)** sections—read both if you can, but focus on the one that speaks to you the most.
- Tear-out **Toolkits** and checklists appear throughout; use them, scribble on them, keep them on the fridge.

Section 1

Anatomy & Basics

Know the Field Before You Play

For Partners (Playbook)

To understand what's changing, you need to know the key players.

- **Ovaries:** the hormone headquarters. They produce estrogen and progesterone—the two main hormones that control cycles, bone strength, mood, and even how blood vessels relax.
- **Uterus:** the muscle that built and shed the monthly lining for years.
- **Brain:** the coach. The hypothalamus and pituitary send signals (FSH and LH) to the ovaries telling them what to do.
- **Adrenal glands:** the substitutes—when ovarian production slows, they step in to make smaller amounts of hormones.

When estrogen levels drop, the whole team feels it: body temperature regulation, sleep cycles, mood balance, and even cholesterol control.

Think of menopause like the off-season: the game doesn't end—you just play differently.

For Women (Huddle)

Estrogen and progesterone are produced mainly in the ovaries. These hormones regulate:

- The menstrual cycle
- Bone growth and calcium absorption
- Cholesterol balance and blood-vessel flexibility
- Brain chemistry that affects mood and memory
- Vaginal and bladder tissue health

During menopause, ovarian hormone production declines gradually until it stops altogether. Without regular estrogen and progesterone:

- The brain reads temperature differently (hot flashes, night sweats).
- Skin and tissues lose some elasticity and moisture.
- Bones lose calcium faster, increasing fracture risk.
- Blood vessels stiffen, raising blood-pressure risk.

These changes don't mean something's wrong—they mean your body is adjusting to a new baseline.

Quick Recap (Take-Home Play)

Team Member	Primary Role	What Changes in Menopause
Brain (Coach)	Sends signals (FSH/LH)	Signals increase to compensate
Ovaries (Players)	Produce estrogen/progesterone	Production decreases, eventually stops
Adrenals (Substitutes)	Make small hormone amounts	Take on partial workload
Bones & Heart (Defense)	Stay strong & flexible	Lose estrogen's protection
Skin, Hair, Vaginal Tissue (Field Conditions)	Stay hydrated & elastic	Become drier, thinner

---

🩺 Anatomy & Basics Toolkit

"Know the Field Before You Play"

Purpose:
Use this page to understand which organs and hormones are the key players during menopause — and how they work together. Bring it to your next visit if you have questions about anatomy or labs.

⚙️ Key Players

System	What It Does	What Changes in Menopause	Notes / Questions
Ovaries	Make estrogen & progesterone	Hormone levels drop; periods stop	
Brain (Hypothalamus & Pituitary)	Send FSH & LH to control cycles	FSH rises as ovaries retire	
Adrenal Glands	Backup source of small hormone amounts	May help smooth transition	
Uterus & Cervix	Build & shed monthly lining	No more cycles; lining thins	
Vagina & Bladder	Elastic tissue for comfort & control	Dryness, urgency, tissue thinning	
Bones & Heart	Depend on estrogen protection	Bone loss ↑ Heart risk ↑	

🧠 **Hormone Cheat Sheet**

Hormone	**Main Job**	**Typical Change**	**My Lab Result / Date**
Estrogen	Controls cycles, bones, mood	Decreases	
Progesterone	Balances estrogen	Decreases	
FSH	Brain signal to ovaries	Increases	
LH	Triggers ovulation	Increases	
Testosterone (Small Amount)	Energy & libido	Slight decrease	

❤ **Reflection Box —** *(Use this space together)*

- ☐ One new thing we learned about how hormones affect health:
- ☐ One question we'll ask at our next visit:
- ☐ One small change we can make to support overall balance (sleep, hydration, etc.):

💡 **Partner Tip**

Understanding biology isn't about memorizing terms — it's about recognizing that hormone shifts drive real, physical changes. Compassion starts with comprehension.

Bring this Toolkit Page to: your next GYN or primary-care visit.

Notes:

Section 2

Stages of Menopause

Reading the Season Schedule

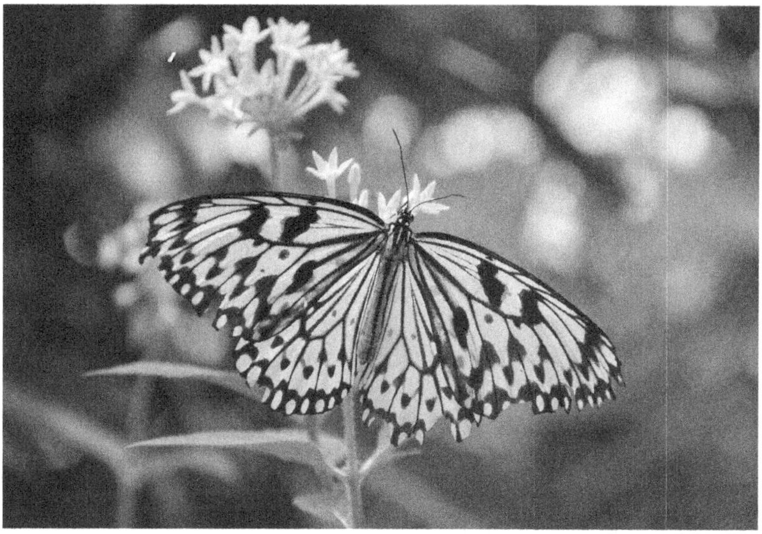

For Partners (Playbook)

If it feels like your wife's moods, sleep, or energy are all over the place, you're not imagining it. Menopause doesn't hit overnight—it's a long transition with clear stages. Think of it as a **multi-season game**, each with its own challenges and adjustments.

Here's the breakdown:

1. **Perimenopause: The Warm-Up and Overtime Period** (Average Age: 40–50)
    - Hormone levels (especially estrogen and progesterone) start to fluctuate unpredictably.
    - Periods may come closer together, farther apart, heavier, lighter, or skip months entirely.
    - Symptoms: hot flashes, mood swings, night sweats, irritability, brain fog, fatigue.
    - She may still **be fertile**, even with irregular cycles.
    - Your job: patience and curiosity, not problem-solving. It's about supporting, not fixing.
2. **Menopause: The Official Time-Out (Average Age: 51)**
    - Defined medically as **12 consecutive months without a menstrual period** (ACOG & UpToDate).
    - The ovaries have officially retired from hormone production.

- Common changes: vaginal dryness, hot flashes, sleep disturbance, changes in libido, slower metabolism.
- It's normal for symptoms to vary—some women have almost none, others struggle daily.
- Your role: normalize the conversation. A sense of humor helps.

3. **Postmenopause: The Long Game (Begins after that 12-month mark)**
    - Hormone levels stay low but steady.
    - Symptoms may ease, but **bone loss and heart risk** become more important to monitor.
    - This is the phase of long-term prevention: exercise, calcium/vitamin D, heart health, and pelvic health matter more than ever.
    - Your role: help maintain good routines—meals, walks, and medical follow-ups.

For Women (Huddle)

Menopause unfolds in phases, not a single event. Each stage has a biological rhythm driven by hormone changes.

1. Perimenopause (The Transition)

- Average onset: age **45–50** (can begin earlier).
- Estrogen and progesterone levels fluctuate, sometimes dramatically.
- You may have heavier or lighter periods, skipped cycles, or PMS-like symptoms that last longer.
- Common experiences include:
    - Hot flashes and night sweats
    - Irregular bleeding
    - Breast tenderness
    - Mood changes
    - Sleep problems
    - Brain fog
    - Changes in libido

💡 *Clinical note:* Ovulation still occurs intermittently—pregnancy is still possible. Continue contraception until you've gone **12 months without a period** (per ACOG).

2. Menopause (The Milestone)

- Medically defined as **12 months without menstruation**, not the day your periods start skipping.
- Average U.S. age: **51**.
- Estrogen levels drop significantly; FSH (the brain's "go" signal) rises sharply.
- Symptoms often peak during this time, lasting from months to several years.

- This is when many women talk with their provider about **hormone therapy (HT)** or non-hormonal symptom management.

---

3. Postmenopause (Life After the Transition)

- Begins **one year after your final period**.
- Periods should not return; any vaginal bleeding now should be evaluated by your medical provider.
- Estrogen remains low and stable.
- Risks shift toward:
  - **Bone loss** (osteopenia or osteoporosis)
  - **Cardiovascular disease**
  - **Genitourinary Syndrome of Menopause (GSM)** – vaginal dryness, urinary urgency or frequency

- Lifestyle and routine medical visits play a major role here.
- Focus on:
  - Strength training, balance, and bone health
  - Heart-healthy nutrition
  - Sexual comfort and connection
  - Preventive care and screenings

Quick Recap: The Three Stages at a Glance

Stage	Avg Age	Hormone Pattern	Key Features	What to Watch For
Perimenopause	40–50	Estrogen & progesterone fluctuate	Irregular cycles, mood swings, hot flashes, night sweats	Fertility still possible, contraception needed
Menopause	~51	Estrogen drops sharply, FSH rises	No periods for 12 months, peak symptoms	Consider hormone therapy discussions
Postmenopause	52+	Low, steady estrogen	Symptoms may ease, bone & heart risk rise	New bleeding must be evaluated

---

🧠 Partner Tip: The Long Season Mindset

Menopause lasts years, not weeks. Symptoms can come and go like streaks in a game—good days, tough days, unexpected overtime. Staying flexible and curious will get you both through it better than any quick fix.

Notes:

🩺 Section 2: Stages of Menopause Toolkit

"Reading the Season Schedule"

Purpose:
Track your symptoms and note where you are in the menopause transition. Use this tool to discuss progress with your provider.

🌑 Menopause Stages Overview

Stage	What's Happening	Common Symptoms	Notes / Questions
Perimenopause	Hormones fluctuate; periods irregular	Hot flashes, mood swings, irregular bleeding	
Menopause	12 months without period	Hot flashes, dryness, fatigue	
Postmenopause	Hormones stay low, steady	Bone & heart changes, GSM symptoms	

🖤 Symptom Tracker

Month	Hot Flashes	Sleep	Mood	Periods	Notes
Jan	☐ Mild ☐ Mod ☐ Severe	☐ Good ☐ Fair ☐ Poor	☐ Stable ☐ Irritable ☐ Sad	☐ Yes ☐ No	
Feb	☐ Mild ☐ Mod ☐ Severe	☐ Good ☐ Fair ☐ Poor	☐ Stable ☐ Irritable ☐ Sad	☐ Yes ☐ No	
Mar	☐ Mild ☐ Mod ☐ Severe	☐ Good ☐ Fair ☐ Poor	☐ Stable ☐ Irritable ☐ Sad	☐ Yes ☐ No	

(Continue as needed.)

💬 Reflection Box

- ☐ I think I'm currently in: ______________________________
- ☐ My top 2 symptoms are: ______________________________
- ☐ I'll bring this tracker to my next visit on: ______________________

💡 Partner Tip

Remember: the stage doesn't define the relationship — it just helps you understand what she's feeling and why.

Notes:

Section 3

Perimenopause, the Transition Years

The Warm-Up, the Overtime, and Every Unexpected Play in Between

For Partners (Playbook)

If you've started noticing that your wife's moods, sleep, or energy seem unpredictable, this is often the first real sign that the "transition years" have started. Perimenopause is like **the longest warm-up in history** — or sometimes like overtime that no one expected to play.

Here's what's happening behind the scenes:

- Her ovaries are **still working**, but not consistently.
- Hormone levels spike and crash unpredictably.
- Estrogen might be high one week (hello, irritability and breast tenderness) and very low the next (cue the night sweats and brain fog).

This hormonal rollercoaster can last several years — and for some women, nearly a decade.

What you'll notice:

- Mood swings that come out of nowhere.
- Forgetfulness or mental fog ("I swear I just had my keys").
- Changes in sleep — waking up hot, restless, or wide awake at 2 a.m.
- Irregular cycles — longer, shorter, or skipped altogether.
- New aches and pains, joint stiffness, or fatigue.

What helps from you:

- Patience beats logic. Don't try to "fix" every symptom.
- Keep the home environment cool at night (literally and emotionally).
- Encourage rest and hydration — both actually help hot flashes.
- Support consistent routines: walks, meals, and laughter.
- Remind her this is temporary — it's a process, not a problem.

For Women (Huddle)

Perimenopause begins when the ovaries start to produce less estrogen and progesterone, but not in a straight line — it's more like a zigzag. These fluctuations affect your menstrual cycle, mood, sleep, and even your metabolism.

Typical Signs You're in Perimenopause (per ACOG & UpToDate):

- Irregular periods — shorter, longer, heavier, or skipped.
- Hot flashes and night sweats.
- Vaginal dryness or discomfort during sex.
- Sleep changes.
- Mood changes (anxiety, irritability, or tearfulness).
- Brain fog or trouble concentrating.
- Breast tenderness or bloating.
- Decreased fertility (but not zero).

💡 *Clinical note:* If you're under age 40 and having these symptoms, your provider may evaluate you for **premature ovarian insufficiency (POI)** or other causes of hormone imbalance.

Medical Evaluation

A provider may recommend:

- **FSH and estradiol levels:** to check hormone fluctuations (though results vary day to day).
- **Thyroid tests:** since thyroid disease can mimic menopause symptoms.
- **Pregnancy test:** to rule out pregnancy if cycles are irregular.
- **Discussion about contraception:** since ovulation can still occur.

Self-Care and Relief Strategies

- **Stay cool:** dress in layers, use a fan at night.
- **Hydrate:** water, not wine, for better symptom control.
- **Eat smart:** plant-based foods, calcium, vitamin D, and fiber.
- **Sleep hygiene:** regular bedtime, limit caffeine, try calming routines.
- **Exercise:** cardio + resistance training help mood, sleep, and bone health.
- **Track your symptoms:** patterns can help guide treatment options.

🔑 **Takeaway**

Perimenopause isn't a single moment — it's a stretch of years where hormones play hide and seek. What matters most is recognizing patterns, communicating openly, and preparing together for the next stage.

💣 Partner + Patient Perspective

Think of this time as a recalibration. Her body is rewriting its playbook — what worked before may not now. The best way to get through it is together: track, talk, and take breaks when needed.

Quick Recap Table

Change	Why It Happens	What It Feels Like	What Helps
Irregular cycles	Hormone fluctuations	Longer, shorter, skipped periods	Track cycles, rule out pregnancy
Hot flashes	Estrogen dips affect brain's thermostat	Sudden heat, flushing, night sweats	Layers, fans, hydration
Mood swings	Shifting estrogen and serotonin	Irritability, anxiety, crying	Sleep, exercise, open conversation
Brain fog	Estrogen affects memory neurotransmitters	Forgetfulness, distraction	Reduce stress, mental breaks
Vaginal dryness	Less estrogen to vaginal tissue	Discomfort with sex	Moisturizers, lubricants
Sleep changes	Hormonal + temperature shifts	Insomnia, restlessness	Cool environment, routine bedtime

🌡 Section 3: Perimenopause Toolkit *"Tracking the Chaos Calmly"*

Purpose:
Use this page to track cycles, triggers, and contraception during the transition years.

💧 Cycle & Symptom Log

Month	Cycle Start Date	Flow (L/M/H)	Hot Flashes	Sleep Quality	Notes
1					
2					
3					
4					
5					
6					
7					
8					
9					
10					
11					
12					

✱ Triggers to Watch

Symptom	Common Trigger	My Pattern
Hot flashes	Alcohol, caffeine, stress	
Mood swings	Sleep loss, sugar intake	
Night sweats	Warm bedroom, stress	
Headaches	Hormone dips, dehydration	
Fatigue	Irregular meals, poor rest	

Contraception Reminder

Pregnancy is still possible until you've gone **12 months without a period.**
Ask your provider about:
☐ IUD ☐ Low-dose pill ☐ Barrier method ☐ Partner vasectomy ☐ Other

Reflection Box

- ☐ The hardest symptom to manage right now: ____________________
- ☐ One habit that helps me most: ____________________
- ☐ Something my partner can do to support me: ____________________

Partner Tip

Support looks like empathy, not solutions. Listen first, help later.

.

Section 4

Emotional & Cognitive Changes

Reading the Defense, Staying Calm When the Game Gets Chaotic

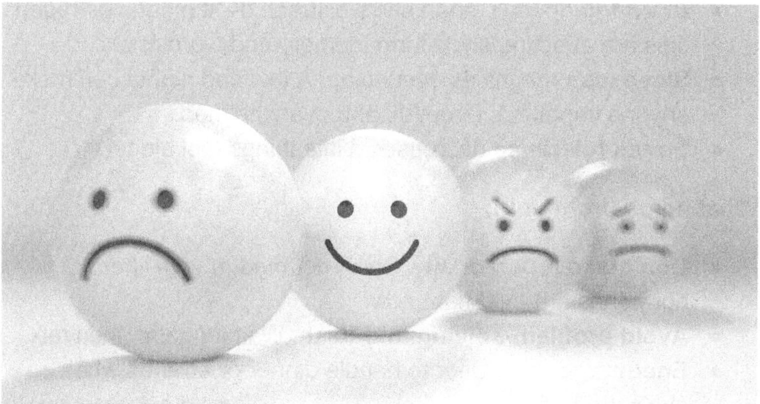

For Partners (Playbook)

If you've found yourself walking into the kitchen one day and getting an icy glare for breathing too loudly, then the next day getting a tearful hug—welcome to **perimenopause defense**. You're not under attack. Her brain chemistry is.

Hormones don't just control physical changes; they shape emotions, sleep, and focus. When estrogen levels swing up and down, neurotransmitters like **serotonin** and **dopamine** swing too. That's why she might go from calm to irritable or weepy without warning.

Here's the inside scoop:

- **Mood swings** aren't personality changes. They're chemical shifts.
- **Brain fog** doesn't mean she's distracted—it means estrogen dips are affecting short-term memory and word recall.
- **Sleep loss** magnifies everything. A few bad nights can make anyone impatient, forgetful, and overwhelmed.
- **Stress tolerance** decreases. Little things feel bigger.

What helps (from you):

- **Don't take it personally.** She's not mad *at you*—her hormones are loud right now.
- **Avoid problem-solving mid-flash.** Wait for calm, then talk.
- **Encourage rest.** Offer to handle dinner or errands when she's drained.
- **Keep humor kind.** Light teasing is fine—mocking isn't.
- **Be consistent.** Predictability makes her feel safe in an unpredictable body.

Think of this phase like facing a new defense—what used to work doesn't anymore. Adjust your plays, stay patient, and keep communicating.

For Women (Huddle)

Your brain is wired with estrogen receptors, which means hormonal fluctuations don't just affect your body—they also affect your mood, memory, and focus. These changes are real and measurable, not "in your head."

What's Happening Biologically (per ACOG & UpToDate)

- **Estrogen regulates serotonin and dopamine**, the same neurotransmitters that stabilize mood.
- As levels fall, **serotonin drops**, leading to irritability, anxiety, or sadness.
- **Sleep disruption** from night sweats or insomnia worsens these symptoms.
- **Brain fog** comes from decreased estrogen support for memory centers (hippocampus).

💡 *Key point:* These symptoms can mimic depression or anxiety, so it's okay—and important—to talk to your provider if you feel persistently sad, unmotivated, or "off."

Common Emotional & Cognitive Symptoms

- Mood swings
- Irritability or anger bursts
- Anxiety or panic
- Sadness or tearfulness
- Difficulty concentrating
- Forgetfulness or "brain fog"
- Feeling less patient or easily overwhelmed

What Helps

- **Routine sleep schedule:** Try to go to bed and wake up at the same time daily.
- **Exercise:** Physical activity releases endorphins and reduces anxiety.
- **Limit alcohol and caffeine:** Both worsen mood swings and sleep.
- **Mindfulness or meditation:** Shown in studies to reduce hot flashes and emotional reactivity.
- **Therapy or counseling:** CBT (cognitive-behavioral therapy) can help manage irritability and insomnia.
- **Medical options:**
    - If mood swings are severe, discuss low-dose SSRIs or SNRIs with your provider (these are non-hormonal and commonly used).
    - Hormone therapy may improve both hot flashes and mood stability when appropriate.

Quick Recap Table

Change	Why It Happens	What It Feels Like	What Helps
Mood swings	Estrogen & serotonin fluctuate	Irritability, tears, short fuse	Sleep, exercise, mindfulness
Anxiety	Neurochemical changes + stress	Racing thoughts, restlessness	Breathing, movement, counseling
Brain fog	Estrogen affects memory centers	Forgetting words, losing focus	Lists, humor, patience
Fatigue	Sleep disruption	Exhaustion, poor coping	Consistent rest, hydration
Sadness	Hormone imbalance	Low motivation, crying	Support, connection, therapy

🧠 Partner + Patient Perspective

You're both on the same team—but you're not playing the same position. She's managing a shifting internal playbook; you're adjusting to the changing rhythm. The best teammates talk between plays, check in, and give grace when the tempo changes.

🗝 Takeaway

Mood and memory changes during menopause are normal, not moral. They don't define her or your relationship. With the right strategies—sleep, humor, support, and medical guidance—you can both keep your heads in the game.

Notes:

🌡 Section 4: Perimenopause Toolkit

"The Transition Years — Tracking the Chaos Calmly"

Purpose:
Use this page to track cycles, triggers, and contraception during the transition years.

💧 Cycle & Symptom Log

Month	Cycle Start Date	Flow (L/M/H)	Hot Flashes	Sleep Quality	Notes
1					
2					
3					
4					
5					
6					

⚙ Triggers to Watch

Symptom	Common Trigger	My Pattern
Hot flashes	Alcohol, caffeine, stress	
Mood swings	Sleep loss, sugar intake	
Night sweats	Warm bedroom, stress	
Headaches	Hormone dips, dehydration	
Fatigue	Irregular meals, poor rest	

Section 5

Lifestyle & Everyday Adjustments

Strength & Conditioning: Building a New Game Plan for Midlife

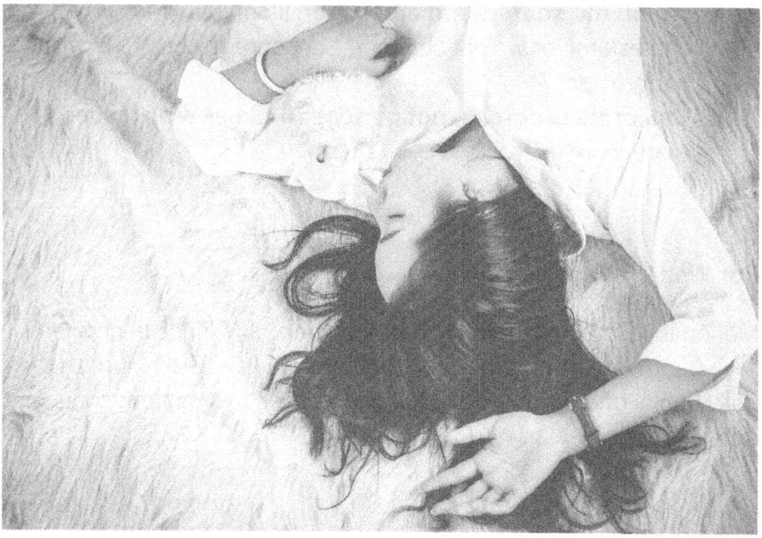

For Partners (Playbook)

Here's the truth: she can't out-exercise hormones, but **how she eats, moves, and rests** now will change how she feels. Your job isn't to become her trainer—it's to **be her teammate**.

When estrogen levels fall, muscle mass, metabolism, and energy often dip too. Bones thin faster, belly fat creeps in, and sleep quality declines. These aren't character flaws; they're biology.

Your role:

- **Join, don't judge.** Walks together beat lectures about diet.
- **Make routines shared.** Schedule workouts, meal prep, and downtime as team activities.
- **Keep movement varied.** Cardio for heart health, weights for bone strength, stretching for flexibility.
- **Watch the scoreboard early.** High blood pressure, rising cholesterol, or weight changes—encourage check-ins with her provider.
- **Celebrate progress, not perfection.** Small wins matter more than "fixes."

For Women (Huddle)

Menopause is a **whole-body recalibration**, and lifestyle choices are your most powerful tools. UpToDate and ACOG emphasize that daily habits often make the biggest difference in symptom control and long-term health.

Nutrition Basics **(general recs-yours may be different)**

- **Calcium:** 1,000–1,200 mg/day for bone protection.
- **Vitamin D:** 600–800 IU/day (ask your provider if labs are low).
- **Protein:** Aim for 20–30 g per meal to preserve muscle.
- **Fiber:** 25+ g daily for heart and gut health.
- **Healthy fats:** Olive oil, avocado, salmon, nuts.
- **Limit:** Added sugars, processed foods, heavy alcohol.

Meal Pattern Goal:

- 3 balanced meals + 1–2 smart snacks.
- Include produce at every meal ("color on the plate").

Try our 5-Day Meal Plan in the Nutrition Toolkit for sample menus and a shopping list.

Movement Matters

Type of Exercise	Target	Why It Helps
Cardio (brisk walk, bike, swim)	150 min/week	Improves heart health & mood
Strength training	2–3× per week	Maintains bone & muscle mass
Flexibility / Balance (yoga, tai chi, pilates)	Daily or alternate days	Reduces injury, improves posture
Pelvic floor exercises	Daily	Supports bladder & sexual health

Even light activity counts—10-minute bouts add up.

🌑 Sleep and Stress Reset

- Keep a consistent bedtime.
- Cool, dark room (65–68°F ideal).
- No screens 1 hour before bed.
- Limit caffeine after noon & alcohol before bed.
- Try 5-minute breathing or mindfulness before lights out.

Stress Management

Menopause stress is cumulative—physical + emotional.

- **Move daily:** exercise lowers cortisol.
- **Mindfulness:** use guided apps or deep breathing.
- **Boundaries:** learn to say no when overloaded.
- **Connection:** maintain social ties; isolation worsens anxiety.

🧩 Partner + Patient Perspective

Think of this chapter as preseason training for the rest of life. The habits you build together now—sleep, movement, balanced meals—set the tone for every future stage.

[Lifestyle Toolkit Page – Nutrition Checklist + 5-Day Meal Plan Summary]

🗝 Takeaway

You can't control hormones, but you can **control your daily rhythm**. Consistent exercise, balanced nutrition, and restorative sleep are the foundation for feeling strong and clear-minded through menopause—and for keeping both of you in the game.

🏋 Section 5: Lifestyle & Everyday Adjustments Toolkit

"Strength & Conditioning: Building Healthy Routines"

Purpose:
Use this page to plan small, daily habits that improve energy, sleep, and long-term health. Simple consistency beats big overhauls.

🍎 Nutrition Tracker

Day	Breakfast	Lunch	Dinner	Snacks / Drinks	Water (cups)
Mon					
Tue					
Wed					
Thur					
Fri					
Sat					
Sun					

💡 *Goal: half your plate fruits/veggies, lean protein, whole grains, and hydration throughout the day.*

Notes:

🚶 Movement Log

Day	Activity	Minutes	Intensity (L/M/H)	How I Felt After
1				
2				
3				
4				
5				

Aim for 150 minutes of moderate exercise weekly (walking, cycling, dancing, swimming).

Reflection Box

- ☐ One habit I'm proud of this week: ______________________
- ☐ One habit to improve next week: ______________________

Partner Tip

Join her! Shared activity keeps motivation up and strengthens connection — even a walk counts as "team training."

Section 6

Surgical & Treatment Induced Menopause

Unexpected Overtime: When the Game Changes Overnight

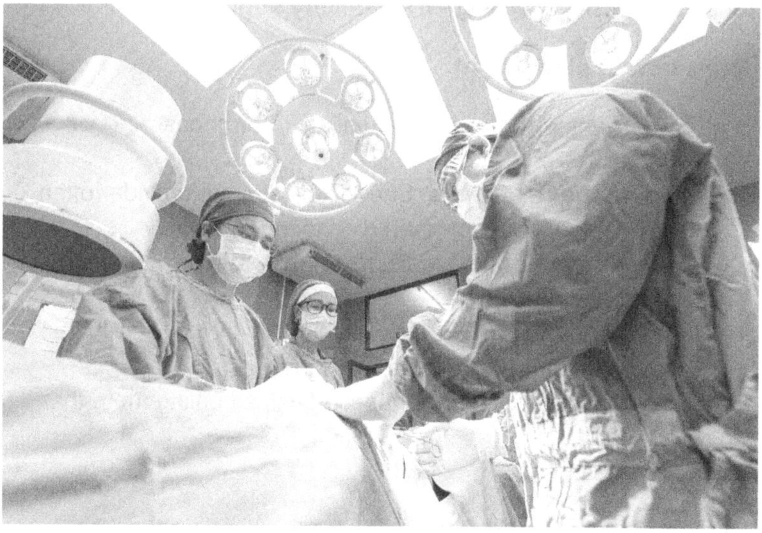

For Partners (Playbook)

Most menopause changes happen gradually over years, but sometimes the game clock speeds up.
When a woman has her ovaries removed (a **bilateral oophorectomy**) or receives certain **cancer or hormone-blocking treatments**, hormone levels drop almost immediately. What usually unfolds over a decade can hit in weeks.

That means:

- Hot flashes appear suddenly and can be intense.
- Sleep, mood, and libido may swing dramatically.
- Recovery from surgery adds physical pain and fatigue to the mix.

Your job now isn't coaching—it's **recovery support.**

Here's how to play it right:

- **Be patient with the pace.** Healing + hormones = unpredictable.
- **Encourage follow-ups.** She'll likely see her provider often for hormone, bone, or heart monitoring.
- **Help with logistics.** Meals, rides, rest, and remembering meds all matter.
- **Avoid minimizing.** Phrases like "At least it's over with fast" sound comforting but can feel dismissive.
- **Stay close.** Emotional connection helps healing more than you realize.

Even if her surgery or treatment was medically necessary, the emotional impact can be huge. Support isn't about fixing—it's about *staying present.*

For Women (Huddle)

When menopause happens because of surgery or medication, your body doesn't get a warm-up—it gets a whistle blow and you're in overtime immediately.

Common Triggers

- **Bilateral oophorectomy:** surgical removal of both ovaries.
- **Chemotherapy or pelvic radiation:** can damage ovarian function.
- **Hormone-blocking medications:** used in breast or ovarian cancer (e.g., tamoxifen, aromatase inhibitors).

What Happens Biologically

- Estrogen and progesterone levels drop sharply.
- Hot flashes, night sweats, vaginal dryness, and mood changes can be stronger than in natural menopause.
- Bone loss and heart-disease risk increase earlier.
- Libido and sexual comfort may change abruptly.

Symptom Management Options

- **Hormone Therapy (HT):** Often considered if there are no cancer-related contraindications. Even low-dose or local estrogen can make a big difference.
- **Non-Hormonal Medications:** SSRIs, SNRIs, gabapentin, or clonidine can reduce hot flashes.
- **Vaginal moisturizers or lubricants:** relieve dryness and pain.
- **Bone protection:** calcium, vitamin D, weight-bearing exercise, or medication if needed.
- **Heart health:** monitor blood pressure, cholesterol, and stay active.

Always review your treatment plan with both your surgeon, oncologist, GYN and/or your primary care provider—each may manage different pieces of recovery.

Emotional Recovery

It's common to grieve the sudden loss of fertility or to feel older overnight. You may experience sadness, anger, or relief—all normal. Consider counseling or a support group, especially if your surgery was tied to cancer or endometriosis.

Partner + Patient Perspective

You can't plan every play, but you can prepare for the next one. Surgical or treatment-induced menopause requires more teamwork, rest, and communication than the natural transition—but the outcome can still be strong, stable, and connected.

Takeaway

When menopause happens suddenly, the goal shifts from "managing change" to **recovering balance**—physically, emotionally, and relationally. With steady support, smart follow-up, and a flexible game plan, you can both adjust to this new normal together.

Notes:

Section 6: Surgical or Treatment-Induced Menopause Toolkit

"Unexpected Overtime: Recovery and Reset"

Purpose:
Use this page to organize your recovery after surgery or hormone-blocking treatment. It's about pacing, healing, and tracking progress.

Recovery Tracker

Date	Symptom or Side Effect	Severity (1–10)	What Helped	Notes for Provider
___				
___				
___				
___				
___				

Medication & Follow-Up Log

Medication	Dose	Purpose	Side Effects	Follow-Up Date
__________				
__________				
__________				
__________				
__________				

♥ Healing Checklist

- ☐ Take prescribed meds as directed
- ☐ Rest more than you think you need
- ☐ Eat protein & stay hydrated
- ☐ Walk daily (short, slow counts)
- ☐ Write down questions for each visit

- ☐ Ask for emotional support — it matters too

Reflection Box

- ☐ Today's biggest victory: ______________________________
- ☐ What I still need help with: ______________________________

Partner Tip

Healing takes time. Offer practical help — meals, rides, notes — and don't rush the process. Presence > pressure. Notes:

Section 7

Heart Health After Menopause

Protecting the Goal: Keeping Your Heart in the Game

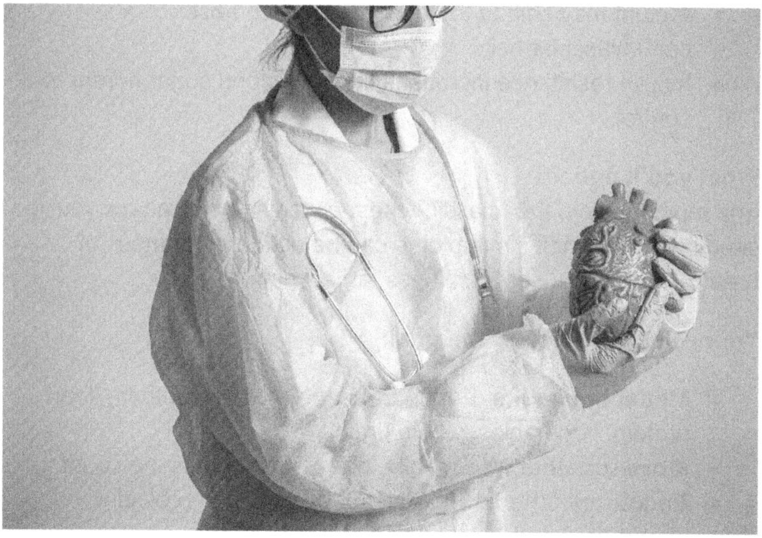

For Partners (Playbook)

Estrogen does more than regulate periods — it protects her heart. When those hormone levels drop, her risk for **heart disease** starts to rise.
Here's the twist: most men know their own cardiac numbers (or at least think they do), but few realize that **heart disease is the number one cause of death in women** — even more than breast cancer.

This is the time to **tighten your defense** as a team.

What happens:

- Estrogen loss increases LDL ("bad") cholesterol and lowers HDL ("good") cholesterol.
- Arteries become stiffer, raising blood pressure.
- Weight may shift to the abdomen, which raises cardiovascular risk.
- Insulin resistance increases, making blood sugar harder to control.

What you'll notice:
She may not have the "classic" chest-clutching heart attack you've seen on TV. Women's symptoms can be quieter: shortness of breath, fatigue, nausea, dizziness, or jaw pain.

Your role in protecting the goal:

- **Model the habits.** Eat heart-healthy foods together—lean protein, vegetables, whole grains.
- **Move together.** Walks, bike rides, even gardening count.
- **Encourage checkups.** Ask her about blood pressure, cholesterol, and glucose goals.
- **Don't ignore fatigue or chest discomfort.** If something feels off, it's worth a visit.
- **Stay positive.** Small, consistent habits prevent big problems.

For Women (Huddle)

After menopause, the drop in estrogen changes how your body handles cholesterol, blood sugar, and blood vessel flexibility. These changes can sneak up quietly but have long-term consequences.

Why Risk Rises After Menopause (per ACOG & ACC):

- Estrogen helps keep arteries flexible. When it drops, arteries stiffen.
- Cholesterol ratios worsen (LDL increases, HDL decreases).
- Blood pressure often rises.
- Weight gain around the middle is common.
- Insulin resistance and prediabetes become more likely.

Know Your Numbers

Test	Healthy Range	When to Check
Blood Pressure	<120/80 mmHg	At least once a year
Total Cholesterol	<200 mg/dL	Every 4–6 years, or yearly if high
LDL (bad cholesterol)	<100 mg/dL	Every 4–6 years, or yearly if high
HDL (good cholesterol)	>50 mg/dL	Every 4–6 years
Triglycerides	<150 mg/dL	Every 4–6 years
A1C (blood sugar)	<5.7%	Every 3 years (more if high risk)
Waist circumference	<35 inches	Regularly

💡 *Tip:* Keep these in your **Heart Health Toolkit**—it's easier to see patterns when they're written down.

Lifestyle Steps That Work

- **Eat for your heart:**
    - Mediterranean-style diet (olive oil, fish, legumes, whole grains).
    - Limit red meat, fried food, and sugary drinks.
    - Add fiber: oats, beans, fruits, veggies.
- **Move daily:**
    - 30 minutes of moderate activity most days.
    - Strength training twice weekly supports metabolism and bone health.
- **Don't smoke.** If you do, get help quitting—it's the fastest way to lower risk.
- **Drink alcohol in moderation:** ≤1 drink/day.
- **Manage stress:** Breathing, stretching, and downtime matter as much as workouts.
- **Sleep:** Poor sleep raises blood pressure and blood sugar. Aim for 7–8 hours.

When to See a Cardiologist

You don't automatically need one, but schedule a consult or ask your PCP for advice if:

- You have **multiple risk factors** (high BP, cholesterol, diabetes, smoking, family history).
- You've had early menopause (<40 years old).
- You notice **chest discomfort, shortness of breath, or new fatigue.**
- You have known heart disease or a strong family history.
- Your primary care provider can coordinate these referrals.

🩺 Partner + Patient Perspective

Heart health is a lifelong game. You don't win it with one big play—you win it with consistent, everyday habits.
This is the perfect stage of life to play defense together: good food, daily movement, and regular medical check-ins are your shared strategy.

🗝️ **Takeaway** Menopause doesn't cause heart disease—but it changes the field. Know your numbers, work as a team, and protect the goal. The same strategies that guard her heart will strengthen yours, too.

Notes:

Notes:

Section 7: Heart Health Tracker Toolkit

"Protecting the Goal: Your Defense Against Heart Disease"

Purpose:
Track vital heart health numbers and lifestyle habits. This helps you and your provider see progress over time.

My Numbers

Metric	My Goal	My Result	Date	Notes
Blood Pressure	<120/80 mmHg			
Total Cholesterol	<200 mg/dL			
LDL (Bad)	<100 mg/dL			
HDL (Good)	>50 mg/dL			
Triglycerides	<150 mg/dL			
A1C (Blood Sugar)	<5.7%			

Daily Heart Habits Checklist

☐ Eat colorful produce daily
☐ Limit fried or processed food
☐ Use olive or avocado oil
☐ Exercise 30 minutes most days
☐ Manage stress (deep breathing, downtime)
☐ Sleep 7–8 hours nightly
☐ Avoid smoking or vaping

💬 Reflection Box

- ☐ One change that's helping my numbers: ______________________________

- ☐ One thing to focus on next: ______________________________

💡 Partner Tip

This isn't just her heart — it's yours too. Making these changes together doubles the benefit and keeps accountability easy.

Notes:

Section 8

Bone Health & Osteoporosis

Strength Training: Building a Better Defense

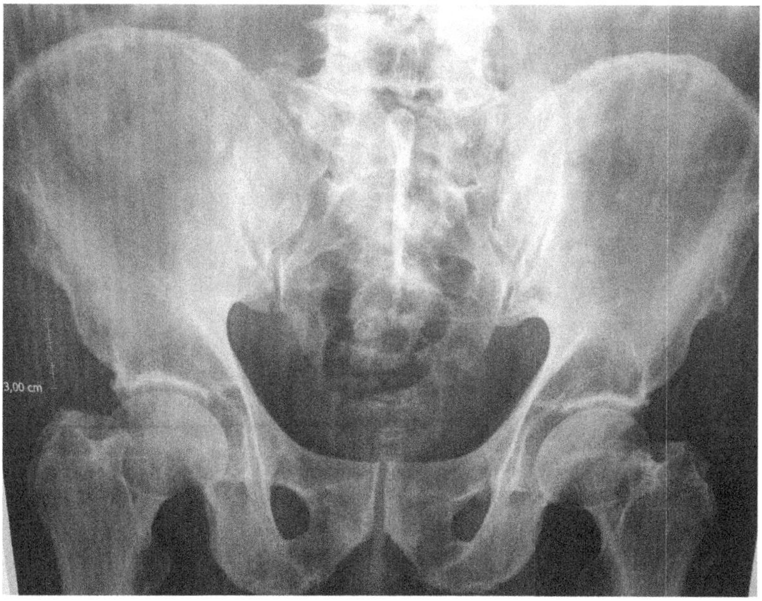

For Partners (Playbook)

When you hear "osteoporosis," you might think of frail bones and hunched backs — but the truth is, bone health is like a **defense line** that starts breaking down quietly after menopause. Estrogen isn't just a reproductive hormone — it's also a key **architect for bone strength**. Once it drops, bones lose density faster, leaving her more vulnerable to fractures.

Here's the play-by-play:

- Bone loss accelerates in the first 5–7 years after menopause.
- The hips, spine, and wrists are the most common fracture zones.
- It's often invisible — no pain until there's a break.

How you can help strengthen the defense:

- **Encourage movement:** walking, light weights, or yoga/pilates are all bone-builders.

- **Be her spotter:** help with home safety (good lighting, no loose rugs, sturdy shoes).

- **Cheer the nutrition changes:** calcium, vitamin D, and protein really matter now.

- **Ask about DEXA scans:** early testing helps catch thinning bones before they break.

- **Be patient:** soreness after new workouts doesn't mean she's fragile — it means she's getting stronger.

Strong bones are built through **daily reps of good habits**, not big moves once a year.

For Women (Huddle)

Estrogen plays a major role in bone metabolism — it helps balance the natural process of bone breakdown (resorption) and rebuilding (formation). After menopause, when estrogen levels fall, this balance tips toward breakdown.

Facts You Should Know (per ACOG & BHOF)

- Women can lose **up to 20% of bone mass** in the first 5–7 years after menopause.
- Osteoporosis affects more women than breast, uterine, and ovarian cancer combined.
- Early screening and prevention make a huge difference.

Bone Health Checklist (applies to most)

- **Calcium:** 1,000–1,200 mg/day (from food or supplements).
- **Vitamin D:** 600–800 IU/day (check your level; many women need more).
- **Protein:** Aim for 20–30 grams per meal to preserve muscle.
- **Caffeine & alcohol:** Too much increases calcium loss.
- **Quit smoking:** Nicotine speeds up bone breakdown.
- **Strength and balance:** Key to preventing falls and fractures.

Notes:

DEXA Scan (Bone Density Test)

- Recommended for all women **≥65 years old**, or earlier if:
  - You've had a fracture after minor injury.
  - You're postmenopausal with risk factors (steroids, family history, small frame, smoking).

- The result is a **T-score**:
  - Normal: above –1.0
  - Osteopenia: –1.0 to –2.5 (low bone mass)
  - Osteoporosis: below –2.5

Bring your results to your **Bone Health Toolkit** for tracking — this makes follow-ups easier.

Medications That May Be Recommended

If lifestyle changes aren't enough, providers may suggest:

- **Bisphosphonates** (alendronate, risedronate): slow bone loss.

- **SERMs** (raloxifene): act like estrogen on bones without affecting breast tissue.

- **Denosumab or teriparatide:** advanced options for severe osteoporosis.

💡 *Always review medication benefits and side effects with your provider — bone strength is important, but every treatment should fit your health history.*

Quick Recap Table

Strategy	Why It Works	Frequency
Weight-bearing exercise	Builds bone density	30 min most days
Strength training	Stimulates bone growth	2–3×/week
Calcium & Vitamin D	Improves bone mineralization	Daily
Fall-proof home	Prevents fractures	Ongoing
DEXA scan	Monitors progress	Every 2–5 years

🧩 Partner + Patient Perspective

Bone health is teamwork: she handles the nutrition and movement, you handle the encouragement and environment. A supportive spotter helps prevent both literal and emotional falls.

🗝 Takeaway

Menopause changes the bone game, but it's one you can win with consistent movement, good nutrition, and regular checkups. You're not just keeping bones strong — you're protecting independence, mobility, and confidence for the long haul.

Notes:

🦴 Section 8: Bone Health Toolkit

"Strength Training: Building a Better Defense"

Purpose:
Track your bone health, calcium and vitamin D intake, and activity goals to protect against fractures and stay strong long term.

📅 Bone Health Tracker

Date	DEXA T-Score	Calcium (mg/day)	Vitamin D (IU/day)	Exercise / Weight Training	Notes

💡 *Ask your provider how often to repeat your DEXA scan — usually every 2–5 years depending on results.*

💪 Bone-Strength Habits Checklist

☐ Weight-bearing activity (walking, dancing, stairs)
☐ Strength training 2–3× per week
☐ Calcium-rich foods daily (yogurt, leafy greens, almonds)
☐ Vitamin D supplement if low
☐ Avoid smoking and excess alcohol
☐ Fall-proof home (good lighting, no loose rugs)

💬 Reflection Box

☐ One bone-friendly food I'll eat more often: ______________________________

☐ My favorite way to stay active: ______________________________

☐ Next DEXA scan due: ______________________________

💡 Partner Tip

Join her on walks or workouts — accountability turns bone health into team health. Notes:

Section 9

Genitourinary Health & Pelvic Floor

Holding the Line: Staying Strong From the Core

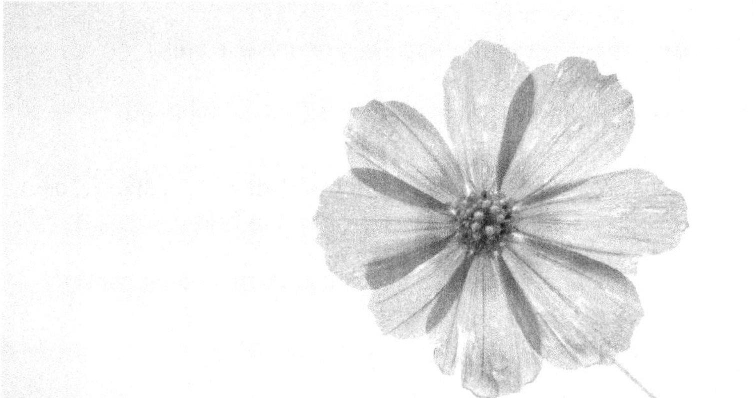

For Partners (Playbook)

This is one of the most uncomfortable topics for couples—but also one of the most important.
When estrogen levels drop, the tissues that support the bladder, urethra, and vagina get thinner and drier. The result can be **leaks, urgency, or discomfort during sex**.

It's called **Genitourinary Syndrome of Menopause (GSM)**—and it's extremely common. It's not about hygiene, and it's not about "aging badly." It's biology.

Here's the game plan:

- **Stay calm and supportive.** These changes are medical, not personal.
- **Encourage her to talk to her provider.** GSM is treatable with safe options.
- **Be patient with intimacy.** Pain or dryness aren't rejection—they're symptoms.
- **Offer solutions, not silence.** A lubricant run to the pharmacy can be an act of love.
- **Help create a bladder-friendly routine.** Limit caffeine, plan restroom stops, and keep humor on the field.

This is a stage where quiet teamwork counts more than highlight plays.

For Women (Huddle)

Estrogen keeps the tissues of your lower urinary tract and vagina thick, elastic, and well-lubricated.
After menopause, that support fades, and symptoms of **GSM** can appear.

Common Symptoms (per ACOG & UpToDate)

- Vaginal dryness, burning, or itching
- Pain with sex (dyspareunia)
- Urinary urgency or frequency
- Stress incontinence (leakage with coughing or laughing)
- Recurrent urinary tract infections
- Sensation of pelvic pressure or "something falling" (prolapse)

💡 *If you notice a bulge, pressure, or new leakage, tell your provider—early treatment is easier and prevents worsening prolapse.*

Understanding the Anatomy

Structure	Role	What Changes After Menopause
Bladder	Stores urine	Loses elasticity; may hold less
Urethra	Carries urine out	Becomes thinner, leading to urgency
Vagina	Provides elasticity & lubrication	Tissues thin, dryness increases
Pelvic Floor Muscles	Support bladder, uterus, rectum	Weaken, causing leakage or prolapse

---

Self-Care & Relief Strategies

- **Vaginal moisturizers:** Use several times a week to restore hydration.
- **Lubricants:** Use during sex—water or silicone-based; avoid scents or warming gels.
- **Pelvic floor exercises:** (See below) strengthen support and reduce leaks.
- **Hydration:** Drink enough water; skipping fluids worsens urgency.
- **Bladder training:** Gradually delay urination to build control.
- **Weight management:** Reduces pressure on the pelvic floor.

Pelvic Floor Exercises (Your Core Defense Line)

Start lying down, then progress to sitting or standing. Consider formal PT/OT with a Pelvic Floor Specialist.

1. **Basic Kegel:** Tighten muscles as if stopping urine; hold 5 sec, relax 5 sec × 10.

2. **Quick Flicks:** Tighten 1 sec / release × 10–20 for sudden urges.

3. **Bridge with Kegel:** Lift hips, engage pelvic floor, lower × 10.

4. **Clamshell:** Side-lying, knees bent, lift top knee × 10 each side.

5. **Wall Sit with Kegel:** Hold contraction 5–10 sec × 5–10 reps.

If leakage or pain continues, ask for a **pelvic floor physical therapy** referral—PTs specialize in this and results are excellent.

When Over-the-Counter Isn't Enough

Talk to your provider about prescription options:

- **Vaginal estrogen** (cream, ring, tablet) – low-dose, acts locally.
- **DHEA suppositories** – rebuild tissue without raising blood estrogen much.
- **Ospemifene (pill)** – improves tissue thickness and reduces pain.
- **Pessary device** – supports pelvic organs if prolapse is significant.

Quick Recap Table

Issue	Why It Happens	What Helps
Dryness	Loss of estrogen	Moisturizers, lubricants, local estrogen
Leaking	Weak pelvic floor	Kegels, PT, bladder training
Urgency	Bladder irritation	Limit caffeine, timed voiding
Pain with sex	Tissue thinning	Lubricants, estrogen therapy
Prolapse	Loss of support	PT, pessary, sometimes surgery

🧩 Partner + Patient Perspective

This is one of the most intimate "team plays" you'll face. It requires honesty, humor, and patience. The goal isn't to get back to "how things used to be"—it's to build a new normal that's comfortable, connected, and confident.

🗝 Takeaway

Menopause affects the entire pelvic system, but it's manageable. With consistent care, communication, and simple exercises, you can both "hold the line" and keep comfort—and confidence—on your side.

Notes:

💧 Section 9: Bladder & Pelvic Floor Toolkit

"Holding the Line: Strength from the Core"

Purpose:
Track bladder habits, pelvic exercises, and symptoms to strengthen control and comfort. Bring this page if seeing a GYN or pelvic floor therapist.

Bladder & Urinary Log

Date	Fluid Intake (cups)	Bathroom Trips (Day/Night)	Urgency (1–5)	Leakage (Y/N)	Notes

Note patterns — frequent urgency or leakage can often improve with exercise or medication.

🧘 Pelvic Floor Exercise Log

Exercise	Reps / Holds	Frequency	Notes
Basic Kegel (5-sec hold)			
Quick Flicks			
Bridge + Kegel			
Wall Sit + Hold			

Reflection Box

- ☐ My biggest challenge right now: ______________________________
- ☐ What helps most: ______________________________
- ☐ Next appointment with pelvic floor PT: ______________________________

Partner Tip

Encourage, don't tease. These exercises take practice — and progress here improves quality of life *and* intimacy. Notes:

Section 10

Menopause & Intimacy

Team Chemistry: Staying Connected on and off the Court

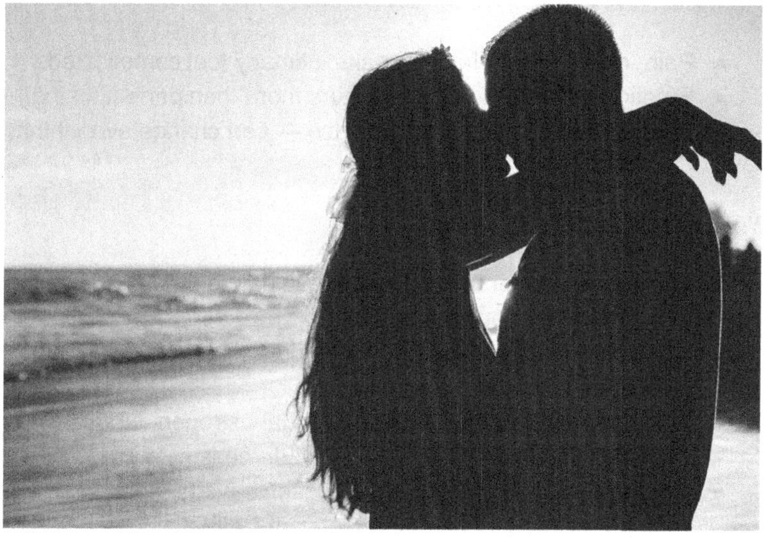

For Partners (Playbook)

Let's be honest — when sex changes, couples notice. But this isn't a story about loss; it's a story about **adjustment**.
During menopause, hormone levels drop, blood flow to the pelvic region decreases, and tissues that used to stretch and self-lubricate don't respond the same way. That can make sex uncomfortable or less spontaneous.

Here's what's **not true:**

- She doesn't want you anymore.
- She's broken or uninterested.
- It's "just mental."

Here's what **is true:**

- Pain, dryness, and fatigue make intimacy feel complicated.
- Emotional connection now matters more than perfect timing.
- The right products — and patience — can change everything.

Your game plan:

- **Don't make it personal.** Pain or avoidance means she's uncomfortable, not rejecting you.
- **Create space for comfort.** A little prep (lighting, timing, lube) goes a long way.
- **Help her talk to her provider.** Vaginal estrogen, lubricants, or moisturizers can relieve pain and dryness safely.
- **Stay involved.** Physical touch doesn't have to mean sex. Hold hands, hug longer, be affectionate without expectations.
- **Mindset shift:** Intimacy after menopause can be *better*, not worse — it just takes teamwork and humor.

For Women (Huddle)

Menopause can affect both physical and emotional aspects of intimacy, but it doesn't have to take sex off the table. Estrogen and testosterone drop, vaginal tissue becomes thinner and drier, and natural lubrication decreases. These are normal biological effects — not personal failings.

Common Physical Changes (per ACOG & ISSWSH)

- Vaginal dryness or tightness
- Pain during sex (dyspareunia)
- Decreased arousal or orgasm intensity
- Slower lubrication
- Weaker pelvic floor tone

💡 *Remember: many of these are reversible with the right care.*

Comfort & Connection Strategies

1. Moisturizers & Lubricants (Over-the-Counter Options)

- **Water-based:** Gentle, safe with condoms/toys; may need reapplication.
- **Silicone-based:** Long-lasting, smooth; ideal for severe dryness.
- **Oil-based:** Natural feel; avoid with condoms (can degrade latex).
- **Hyaluronic acid or Vitamin E–based moisturizers:** Long-term tissue hydration, used several times a week.

💡 *Avoid warming or scented products—they often cause irritation.*

---

2. Prescription Treatments (Discuss with Your Provider)

- **Vaginal Estrogen (cream, tablet, or ring):** Restores elasticity and moisture.
- **DHEA suppositories:** Promote tissue repair without increasing systemic estrogen.
- **Ospemifene (oral):** Non-hormonal, improves vaginal comfort and sexual function.

These are safe for most women but should be individualized—especially if there's a history of cancer, blood clots, or other health concerns.

---

3. Emotional Connection & Rebuilding Desire

- **Shift the focus:** Make intimacy broader than intercourse.
- **Communicate openly:** Tell your partner what feels good and what doesn't.
- **Schedule intimacy:** Spontaneity is great, but planning helps reduce anxiety.
- **Mind-body work:** Yoga, pelvic floor therapy, and mindfulness can reconnect you with your body.
- **Therapy or sex counseling:** A trained therapist can guide you through physical or emotional barriers.

Quick Recap Table

Concern	Why It Happens	What Helps
Vaginal dryness	Low estrogen	Moisturizers, lubricants, vaginal estrogen
Pain with sex	Thinner tissue, low lubrication	OTC or prescription therapy
Low desire	Hormonal + stress + fatigue	Communication, therapy, shared relaxation
Discomfort with intimacy	Physical or emotional changes	Patience, humor, new approaches

---

🧩 Partner + Patient Perspective

Think of this as working on **team chemistry**, not performance stats. It's about listening, adjusting, and keeping connection alive in all forms.
Sometimes the most intimate thing you can do is show understanding instead of urgency.

🗝 Takeaway

Menopause can change intimacy, but it doesn't erase it. With the right tools, communication, and mutual patience, couples often find this stage brings deeper closeness than ever before.

Notes:

💞 Section 10: Sexual Health Comfort Toolkit

"Team Chemistry: Staying Connected On and Off the Court"

Purpose:
Track comfort, products, and strategies that make intimacy easier and more enjoyable. Share this page with your provider if needed.

💧 Comfort & Moisture Log

Date	Product Used	Type (Moisturizer/Lubricant/Prescription)	Relief (1–5)	Notes

💡 *Regular moisturizers hydrate tissue long term; lubricants help in the moment.*

🛒 My Comfort Toolkit

Product Category	Examples	Tried? (Y/N)	Notes
Water-based lubricant	KY Jelly, Astroglide, Good Clean Love		
Silicone-based lubricant	Pjur, Uberlube, Replens Silky		
Moisturizer (hyaluronic acid / Vitamin E)	Hyalo GYN, Revaree		
Local estrogen (cream, ring, tablet)	Estrace, Vagifem, Estring		
DHEA or Ospemifene	Insert or pill, by Rx		

Reflection Box

- ☐ What's working best for me: ______________________________
- ☐ What I'd like to ask my provider about: ______________________________
- ☐ One way my partner helps keep connection strong: ______________
  ____
  ____

Partner Tip

Intimacy is about comfort and confidence. Focus on laughter, patience, and communication — not perfection. Notes:

Section 11

Communication & Connection

Gameplan for Two: Keeping the Team Strong

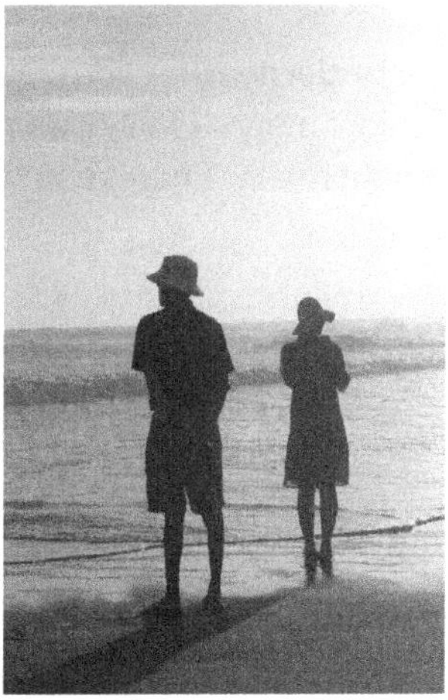

For Partners (Playbook)

No one wins a championship without talking between plays. Menopause isn't just a hormone shift—it's a communication test. You can't read her mind, and she can't always predict how she'll feel. The trick is to keep talking even when things get uncomfortable.

Here's how to stay connected when the signals get crossed:

1. **Lead with curiosity, not correction.**
   - Ask, "How can I help?" instead of "What's wrong?"
   - Sometimes she just wants to vent, not troubleshoot.

2. **Stay calm under pressure.**
   - If she's irritated, it's not always about you.
   - Step back, breathe, and give space when needed.

3. **Listen for what's underneath.**
   - "I'm tired" might mean "I feel overwhelmed."
   - "I'm fine" might mean "I need a hug but don't know how to ask."

4. **Show up outside the crisis.**
   - Little gestures—a note, making coffee, handling chores—score quiet points that matter.

5. **Keep humor kind.**
   - Laugh together, never at her expense.
   - Shared laughter lowers stress and strengthens your bond.

The big idea: You're not trying to *fix* menopause; you're trying to *stay in rhythm*. Talk, listen, and keep your cool.

For Women (Huddle)

Menopause can shake confidence and communication on both sides. Between hot flashes, sleep loss, and emotional swings, it's easy to pull back instead of reaching out. But connection is medicine—emotionally and physically.

Ways to communicate clearly and kindly:

1. **Use "I" statements.**
   - "I'm feeling anxious tonight" lands better than "You're stressing me out."
   - It invites teamwork instead of blame.

2. **Set expectations early.**
   - If you need quiet time, say so.
   - If you want help, ask directly—partners can't read between hormonal lines.

3. **Acknowledge what's changing.**
   - "I'm not sleeping, so I'm shorter-tempered than usual."
   - Owning it keeps empathy alive.

4. **Remember self-image.**
   - Hormone changes, weight shifts, and body differences can affect confidence.
   - Share those feelings instead of hiding them—vulnerability builds closeness.

5. **Keep connection simple.**
   - Shared meals, walks, and inside jokes keep emotional muscle strong.

💡 *If conversation keeps looping into frustration, consider counseling or couples therapy—many providers specialize in midlife transitions.*

Love Languages: Knowing Each Other's Playbook (from Gary Chapman's *The 5 Love Languages*)

Love Language	What It Means	Example in Midlife
Words of Affirmation	Feeling valued through words	"I appreciate everything you do."
Acts of Service	Help = love	Taking over errands when she's exhausted
Quality Time	Full attention matters	Unplugged dinner or evening walk
Gifts	Thoughtful tokens	Favorite snack, new journal
Physical Touch	Reassurance through contact	Hug, hand on shoulder, cuddle night

Quick Recap Table

Skill	Why It Matters	How to Practice
Listening	Reduces conflict	Eye contact, no interruptions
Validation	Builds trust	"That sounds hard, I get it."
Humor	Diffuses tension	Share, don't mock
Vulnerability	Deepens intimacy	Admit fears or needs
Teamwork	Strengthens bond	Share chores, decisions, and wins

🧩 Partner + Patient Perspective

Every great team survives a rough season because they keep showing up. Communication isn't about perfection—it's about staying engaged, even when the playbook changes daily. The goal is progress, not perfection.

🗝 Takeaway

Menopause tests patience, empathy, and timing—but it can also deepen partnership. Keep talking, keep laughing, and remember: you're on the same team, chasing the same win—connection that lasts.

Notes:

💬 Section 11: Communication & Connection Toolkit

"Game Plan for Two: Keeping the Team Strong"

Purpose:
Use these questions to start open conversations and strengthen teamwork. Fill them out privately first, then compare notes together.

🧍 For Husbands — Questions to Ask (and Listen To)

Question	Check if You've Asked	Her Answer / Notes
What's been hardest for you lately?	☐	
Is there something I do that makes bad days better?	☐	
What could I do differently when you're overwhelmed?	☐	
Do you want me to give advice, or just listen?	☐	
How can I support you with appointments or symptoms?	☐	
Are there days when space helps more than company?	☐	
What makes you feel most loved right now?	☐	
How can I make home feel calmer?	☐	
Would you like me to learn more about menopause with you?	☐	
What would help us laugh more together?	☐	

💡 *Goal: ask one question at a time—don't rapid-fire. Listen fully before responding.*

🚶 For Wives — Questions to Ask (and Share)

Question	Check if You've Asked	His Answer / Notes
How are you feeling about these changes?	☐	
Is there something I do that makes you feel shut out?	☐	
How can I explain what's happening without sounding defensive?	☐	
Do you want details, or just headlines?	☐	
What's been hardest for you to understand?	☐	
How can I show appreciation when you help?	☐	
What kind of downtime helps you reset?	☐	
How do you best like to connect—talking, touch, humor, quiet?	☐	
Is there anything you miss that we can rebuild together?	☐	
What's one fun thing we should plan soon?	☐	

💡 *These questions are about teamwork, not blame. Curiosity = connection.*

🖤 Love Language Circles

Circle your top two: Partner–

Words

Acts

Time

Gifts

Touch

Circle your top two: Woman

Words

Acts

Time

Gifts

Touch

Compare circles—then do one small gesture from each other's list this week.

💬 Reflection Box

- ☐ One new thing I learned about you: ______________________________
- ☐ One thing I'll try this week: ______________________________________

💡 Partner Tip

Talk when both of you are rested and calm—never mid-flash or mid-argument.

Notes:

Section 12

Hormone Therapy

Strategic Substitutions: When the Team Needs Extra Support

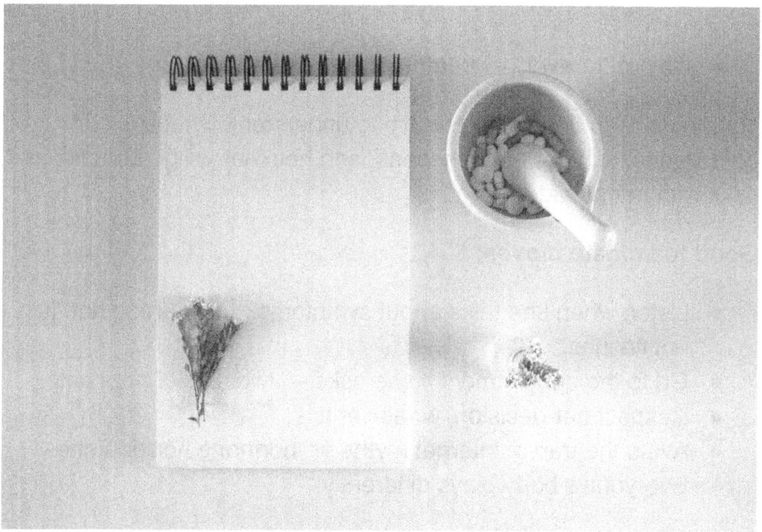

For Partners (Playbook)

Sometimes a team needs a substitute player. Hormone therapy (HT) is exactly that — a way to replace what the body has stopped producing. It doesn't reverse menopause, but it can **reduce hot flashes, improve sleep, protect bone health, and help comfort and mood.**

You'll probably hear mixed opinions about HT. Here's what you need to know:

- It's **safe and effective for many women** when started near the time of menopause.

- The decision is **personal and medical** — it depends on age, health history, and symptoms.

- It's not "forever" — treatment is reviewed regularly.

Your job isn't to decide for her. It's to understand what she's considering, support her questions, and help her weigh benefits and risks with her provider.

Good teammate moves:

- Listen when she talks about symptoms; they're real, not "just hot flashes."
- Go to the appointment if she asks — two sets of ears help.
- Respect her decision, whatever it is.
- Avoid the trap of internet myths or "hormone horror stories." Everyone's body plays differently.

For Women (Huddle)

Hormone therapy replaces the estrogen (and sometimes progesterone) your ovaries no longer make. According to **ACOG** and **UpToDate**, it's still the **most effective treatment** for hot flashes, night sweats, and vaginal dryness.

Types of Hormone Therapy

Type	What It Is	Who It's For	Notes
Systemic Estrogen (pills, patches, gels, sprays)	Replaces estrogen throughout the body	Women with moderate–severe symptoms like hot flashes	Reduces symptoms, protects bones
Combined Estrogen + Progesterone	Estrogen + progestin	Women who still have a uterus	Progesterone protects uterus lining from overgrowth
Vaginal Estrogen (local)	Creams, rings, tablets	Women with vaginal dryness only	Acts locally, very low absorption
Non-Hormonal Alternatives	SSRIs, SNRIs, others	Women who can't take hormones	Reduce hot flashes and mood symptoms

Potential Benefits of Hormone Therapy

- Reduces hot flashes and night sweats
- Improves sleep and quality of life
- Restores some vaginal tissue and helps comfort
- Helps prevent bone loss and fractures
- May improve skin elasticity and joint comfort

Risks and Precautions

Modern hormone therapy is **much safer** than older regimens, but it still requires personalized care. Please discuss with your provider.

Avoid or use caution if you have:

- History of breast or uterine cancer
- Blood clots or stroke
- Uncontrolled high blood pressure
- Liver disease

💡 *Most risks depend on timing and dose.* Starting HT **before age 60 or within 10 years of menopause** is usually considered safest. (ACOG & NAMS)

Choosing the Right Form

Your provider will tailor therapy to your needs:

- **Pills:** easy but slightly higher clot risk.
- **Patches/Gels/Sprays:** steady absorption, lower clot risk.
- **Rings/Tablets:** for vaginal symptoms only.

Regular follow-ups check blood pressure, weight, and breast health.

Tapering or Stopping

Hormone therapy isn't "one and done." Some women use it for a few years, others longer. Providers re-evaluate yearly to decide whether to continue, taper, or stop. If stopped suddenly, symptoms may return briefly — like a rebound in overtime.

Quick Recap Table

Goal	Best Option	Notes
Hot flashes, night sweats	Systemic estrogen	Add progesterone if uterus intact
Vaginal dryness only	Local estrogen	Minimal systemic absorption
Bone health	Systemic estrogen	Especially helpful early in menopause
Can't take hormones	Non-hormonal meds	Discuss SSRIs/SNRIs with provider

---

🧩 Partner + Patient Perspective

Hormone therapy is about **quality of life**, not vanity. When symptoms calm down, sleep returns, and energy rebounds, everyone benefits. The key is staying informed, monitoring health, and trusting the plan you build with your provider.

🗝 Takeaway

Hormone therapy isn't a miracle—it's a medical option that can make menopause more livable. Like any good substitution, it works best with strategy, communication, and regular check-ins.

Notes:

💊 Section 12: Hormone Therapy Toolkit

"Strategic Substitutions: Tracking What Works"

Purpose:
Record treatment plans, benefits, and questions for your provider.

🩺 My Hormone Therapy Plan

Type (Pill/Patch/Cream)	Dose	Start Date	Benefits	Side Effects / Notes

---

📓 Follow-Up & Monitoring

Appointment Date	Labs or Imaging	Provider Notes	Next Check

Questions for My Provider

☐ What form and dose are best for me?
☐ What side effects should I watch for?
☐ How often will we re-evaluate?
☐ Can I combine this with non-hormonal treatments?
☐ How long should I stay on therapy?

Reflection Box

☐ How I'm feeling since starting treatment: ____________________________

☐ What I'll discuss at my next visit: ____________________________________

Partner Tip

Help her stay consistent—reminders and encouragement matter more than opinions about the treatment itself.
Notes:

Section 13

Non-Hormonal Options

Alternative Plays: Different Routes to the Same Goal

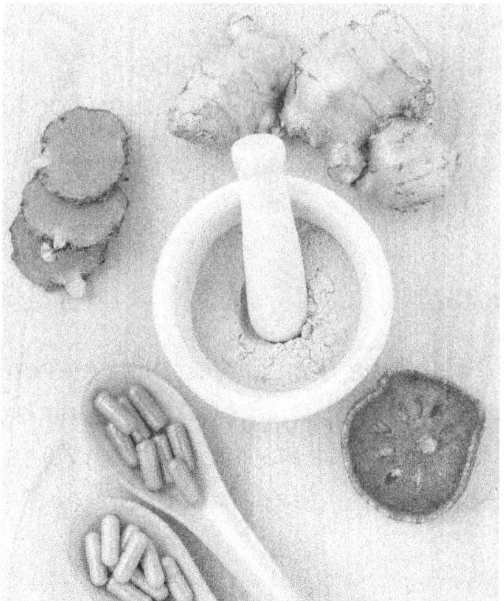

For Partners (Playbook)

Hormone therapy isn't for everyone. Some women can't take it because of cancer history, blood clots, or personal choice. But that doesn't mean there aren't **good plays left on the board**.

Non-hormonal options can still **relieve hot flashes, improve sleep, balance mood, and ease vaginal dryness**.
They just use different pathways — through the brain, nerves, and lifestyle.

Your role in this play:

- Be supportive, not skeptical. These aren't "lesser" options—they're smart alternatives.
- Encourage her to stay consistent; many take a few weeks to show results.
- Keep track of what helps and what doesn't.
- Remember: you're playing for *long-term comfort*, not quick fixes.

For Women (Huddle)

If hormone therapy isn't the right fit, you still have **effective non-hormonal options** supported by **ACOG** and **UpToDate** research. These fall into three main categories: **prescription medications, lifestyle changes, and supplements**.

Prescription Medications

Medication Type	Examples	What They Help	Notes
SSRIs / SNRIs (antidepressants)	Paroxetine, Venlafaxine, Escitalopram	Hot flashes, mood changes, sleep	Non-hormonal; may help within 1–2 weeks
Gabapentin	Neurontin	Night sweats, sleep improvement	Best taken at bedtime; mild dizziness possible
Clonidine	Catapres	Hot flashes, blood pressure	May lower BP too much in some people
Fezolinetant *(new FDA-approved)*	Veozah	Moderate to severe hot flashes	Targets the brain's heat-control center, not hormones

💡 *These work by calming the brain's "thermostat," not replacing hormones.*

Lifestyle Adjustments (Your Daily Game Plan)

Even small changes add up:

- **Keep the cool advantage:** Use layers, fans, breathable bedding.
- **Exercise regularly:** Improves mood, energy, and sleep.
- **Limit triggers:** Caffeine, alcohol, and spicy foods can worsen hot flashes.

- **Manage stress:** Deep breathing, yoga, or mindfulness lower symptom intensity.
- **Stay hydrated:** Keeps temperature stable and reduces headaches.

Supplements & Herbal Options

Here's the reality: most over-the-counter "menopause miracles" aren't backed by solid science. But a few have some research behind them.

Supplement	Claimed Benefit	What We Know	Safety Tip
Black Cohosh	Reduces hot flashes	Mixed results; may help some women short-term	Avoid if liver disease or on meds that go thru the liver
Soy Isoflavones	Plant estrogen mimic	Mild benefit for hot flashes in some	Avoid with estrogen-sensitive cancers unless cleared
Flaxseed	Mild symptom relief, heart health	May help hot flashes, adds fiber	Safe; start gradually for digestion
Evening Primrose Oil	Hormone balance	Studies show little benefit	May cause headache or nausea
St. John's Wort	Mood improvement	May help mild depression	Strong drug interactions—ask provider

Vitamin E	Mild hot flash relief	Modest evidence; generally safe	Keep dose <400 IU daily

👉 *Always tell your provider about any supplements—"natural" doesn't always mean safe.*

Vaginal Comfort Without Hormones

- **Hyaluronic acid moisturizers** (like Replens or Hyalo GYN): retain moisture for days.
- **Silicone-based lubricants:** long-lasting comfort during intimacy.
- **Regular use:** 2–3x per week, not just before sex.

Combining Approaches

Many women find best results with a mix:

- A non-hormonal prescription for hot flashes
- Daily lifestyle changes
- Local OTC treatments for dryness
- Stress reduction or counseling for mood

Menopause care is like a team sport — no single player wins the game, but the right combination does.

Quick Recap Table

Category	Helps Most With	Key Benefit	Provider Role
Medications (SSRIs, Gabapentin, etc.)	Hot flashes, sleep, mood	Quick relief, non-hormonal	Prescribe and monitor side effects
Lifestyle	All-around health	Improves energy, mood, heart	Guide realistic goals
Supplements	Mild hot flashes, mood	Natural options for mild symptoms	Check safety interactions
Vaginal Moisturizers	Dryness, comfort	Local relief, OTC	Recommend safe products

---

🧩 Partner + Patient Perspective

You don't have to run only one play. Menopause management is flexible — different combinations work for different women. The best results come from teamwork: track what helps, celebrate small wins, and stay consistent.

🗝 Takeaway

Menopause isn't a one-size-fits-all journey. Whether it's prescription, nutrition, movement, or mindfulness, the goal is comfort, energy, and confidence. The right mix of plays keeps everyone in the game.

🌿 Section 13: Non-Hormonal Options Toolkit

"Alternative Plays: Tracking What Else Works"

Purpose: Use this tracker to log non-hormonal medications, supplements, and lifestyle strategies.

▇ Medication & Supplement Log

Name	Dose	Purpose	Started	Benefit (1–5)	Side Effects / Notes

💡 *Include vitamins, herbal products, and over-the-counter remedies so your provider has the full picture.*

🧘 Lifestyle Strategies Tracker

Habit	Frequency	How It Helps	Keep / Adjust
Exercise			
Sleep routine			
Mindfulness			
Diet changes			
Hydration			

💬 Reflection Box

- ☐ What's been most helpful so far: ______________________________
- ☐ One thing I want to ask my provider about: ______________________

🌹 Partner Tip

Support consistency: the success of non-hormonal options depends on routine, not luck.

Section 14

Preparing for Your First Visit

Pregame Strategy: Showing Up Ready to Win

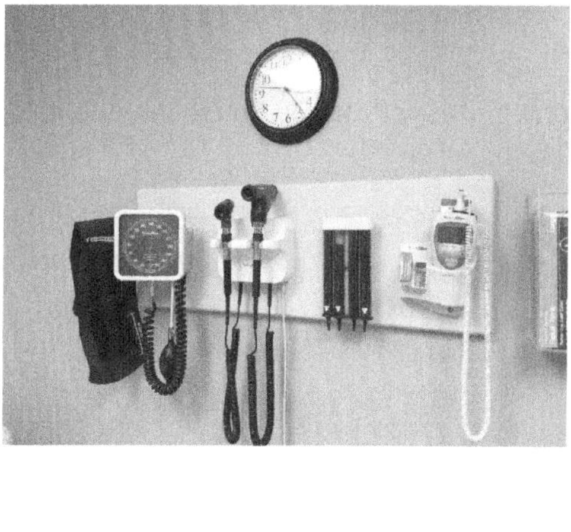

For Partners (Playbook)

When it comes to menopause, the doctor's visit is more than a checkup — it's **game planning.**
Your partner's provider will help figure out what's happening hormonally, rule out other causes of symptoms, and tailor treatment options. You can be part of the strategy without taking over the playbook.

How to be a good teammate:

- Offer to go along if she wants backup.
- Help her write down symptoms or questions ahead of time — memory can blur in the office.
- Stay supportive if she feels emotional or unheard.
- Respect that some topics may stay between her and the provider.

The goal is confidence, not control. You're there to help her feel heard, not to do the talking.

For Women (Huddle)

Being prepared for your menopause visit can make all the difference. Your provider can only treat what they know — and the more specific you are, the better your care plan will be.

Here's your **pregame checklist** for the appointment:

1. Bring Your Health Stats

- Current medications, vitamins, and supplements
- Blood pressure readings (if you monitor at home)
- Recent labs or imaging reports (if available)
- List of chronic conditions (e.g., hypertension, diabetes, thyroid disease)

2. Track Your Symptoms

Write down what you've noticed over the last few months.

Symptom	When It Started	How Often	How It Affects You
Hot flashes / night sweats			
Mood swings / anxiety			
Sleep trouble			
Irregular periods / bleeding			
Vaginal dryness or pain			
Urinary urgency or leakage			
Fatigue or brain fog			
Weight changes			

Bring this to the visit — it saves time and gives your provider a clear picture.

3. Know Your Family History

Tell your provider about any **first-degree relatives** (mother, sisters, daughters) with:

- Breast, ovarian, or uterine cancer
- Blood clots or stroke
- Early menopause or infertility
- Osteoporosis or hip fractures
- Heart disease

This helps guide safe treatment options.

---

4. Common Questions to Ask Your Provider

1. Am I in perimenopause or menopause?
2. Are there labs or tests I should have?
3. What can I do to manage hot flashes or night sweats?
4. Is hormone therapy right for me?
5. What are non-hormonal options if I can't take hormones?

6. Should I be screened for bone loss or heart disease?

7. How often should I have pelvic exams or Pap smears now?

8. When should I worry about unexpected bleeding?

9. Are there lifestyle changes that can make symptoms easier?

10. What local or online support resources do you recommend?

5. Partner's Role in the Visit

If he comes with you, let him know what you want:

- Do you want him to listen quietly or take notes?
- Are there parts of the discussion you'd rather keep private?
- Would you like help remembering instructions afterward?

Clear roles make the appointment smoother and more productive.

Quick Recap Table

Step	Why It Matters	Tip
Track symptoms	Gives clear data	Use your Toolkit log
List medications	Avoids interactions	Include OTC and herbs
Know family history	Guides safe treatment	Note cancers, heart disease, clots
Prepare questions	Keeps you focused	Write down top 3 priorities
Partner support	Reduces stress	Agree on his role before the visit

---

🧩 Partner + Patient Perspective

Think of the office visit as a team huddle with your provider as the coach. Preparation means better decisions, fewer surprises, and faster progress toward comfort and balance.

🗝 Takeaway

Showing up prepared turns a stressful visit into a confident, informed conversation. The more you plan together, the better your provider can help design the winning strategy for your next stage of life. Notes:

🩺 Section 14: Doctor Visit Toolkit

"Pregame Strategy: Showing Up Ready to Win"

Purpose: Use this checklist before and after each appointment to make sure all your questions and updates are covered. Bring this page with you or take a photo of it on your phone.

📋 Before the Visit

Task	Done (✓)	Notes
Write down top 3 concerns or symptoms	☐	
Update medication & supplement list	☐	
Record recent BP, weight, and labs	☐	
Note family history changes	☐	
Bring symptom tracker or toolkit pages	☐	
Write down new questions	☐	

💬 Questions to Ask

Question	Answer / Notes
Am I in perimenopause or menopause?	
What treatments fit my health history?	
What labs or screenings do I need?	
Are my symptoms typical or concerning?	
What lifestyle changes would help most?	
When should I follow up next?	

After the Visit

Task	Done (✓)	Notes
Fill prescriptions & set reminders	☐	
Schedule imaging, labs, or follow-ups	☐	
Update partner/family on changes	☐	
Write 1–2 takeaways from today	☐	

Reflection Box

- ☐ My next appointment date: ______________________________
- ☐ One thing that surprised me today: _____________________
- ☐ What I'll do differently this week: _____________________

Partner Tip

Ask, "How did it go?"—not, "What did they say?" Listening for emotions helps more than decoding the details.

Section 15

Abnormal or Unexpected Bleeding

Flag on the Play: When to Call for a Review

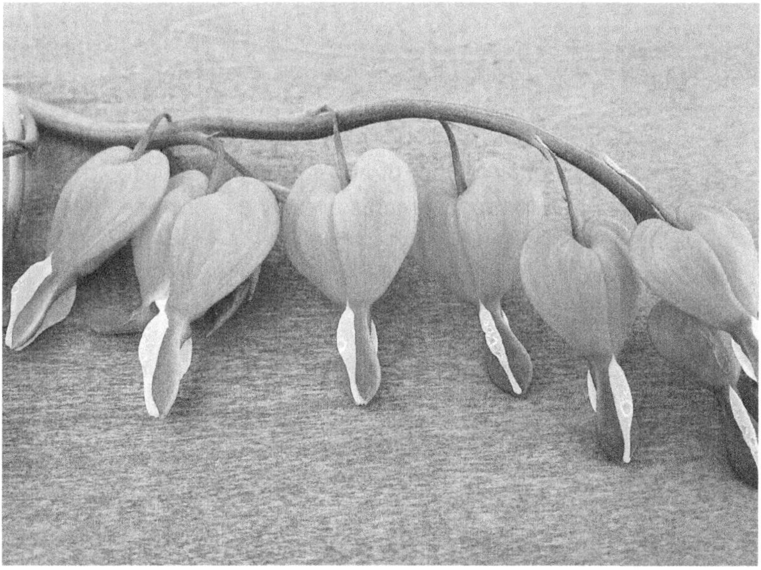

For Partners (Playbook)

Here's one of the most confusing things about menopause: bleeding doesn't always follow the rules.
During perimenopause, cycles can be irregular for years — long gaps, heavy months, or spotting in between. That's normal. But once she's officially in menopause (no periods for 12 months), **any new vaginal bleeding is a red flag** — not an emergency, but something her provider needs to evaluate.

Why it matters:

- Postmenopausal bleeding can be caused by many things — most are benign (like vaginal dryness or a fragile lining).
- Occasionally, it signals something that needs treatment, such as **polyps, fibroids, or uterine lining changes**.
- The sooner it's checked, the easier it is to address.

Your role:

- Stay calm — don't panic or downplay it.
- Encourage her to call her provider promptly.
- Offer support for appointments or testing — it's often just an ultrasound or office biopsy.
- Don't say, "It's probably nothing." Say, "Let's get it checked to be safe."

Catching issues early is like challenging a bad call — better to review it right away than ignore it and regret it later.

For Women (Huddle)

Bleeding after menopause is never "normal," but it's often **not dangerous**. It's your body's way of asking for a quick evaluation.

Common Causes of Postmenopausal Bleeding (per ACOG & UpToDate)

Cause	What It Means	Treatment
Vaginal atrophy (GSM)	Thinner, drier tissue that bleeds easily	Vaginal estrogen, moisturizers
Endometrial or cervical polyps	Benign growths in uterus or cervix	Office removal
Fibroids (leiomyomas)	Noncancerous muscle growths	Observation or minor surgery
Endometrial hyperplasia	Thickened uterine lining	Hormone therapy or biopsy follow-up
Endometrial cancer	Abnormal cells in uterine lining	Surgery, often curable when found early
Medications	Blood thinners, HRT changes, supplements	Medication review and adjustment

During Perimenopause (Still Cycling)

Bleeding may vary — heavier, lighter, skipped months — because hormones rise and fall unpredictably.

Call your provider if:

- Periods last longer than 8 days.
- You soak through a pad/tampon every hour for 2+ hours.
- You pass large clots or feel dizzy/lightheaded.
- Bleeding occurs after sex.

After Menopause (No Periods for 12 Months)

Any bleeding — even light spotting — should be evaluated. Your provider may recommend:

1. **Pelvic exam:** to check vaginal and cervical tissue.
2. **Transvaginal ultrasound:** measures uterine lining thickness.
3. **Endometrial biopsy:** simple office test to sample uterine cells.
4. **Pap smear or cervical screening:** if due.

Other Possible Causes

- New blood thinners (aspirin, warfarin, apixaban)
- Herbal supplements like ginkgo or high-dose fish oil
- HRT dose changes
- Vaginal trauma or dryness

💡 *Tip:* Track when and how much bleeding occurs—it helps your provider pinpoint the cause faster.

Preventive Screenings & Ongoing Gynecologic Care

Even after menopause, routine GYN visits are still important.

Screening	Frequency (per ACOG)	Notes
Pelvic exam	Every 1–2 years	May adjust based on risk
Pap test (cervical cancer)	Every 3–5 years until age 65 (if normal history)	May stop if no abnormal results for 10 years
Mammogram	Every 1–2 years (per ACS/USPSTF)	Continue as long as healthy
DEXA (bone density)	At or after age 65, or earlier with risk factors	Track in Bone Health Toolkit
Colonoscopy	Every 10 years (or stool-based yearly tests)	Preventive, not menopause-specific

Quick Recap Table

Stage	Normal Bleeding	Call Your Provider If...
Perimenopause	Irregular, but within reason	Periods too heavy, too long, or between cycles
Menopause/ Postmenopause	None	Any spotting or flow after 12 months period-free

---

🧩 Partner + Patient Perspective

It's easy to assume "a little bleeding" isn't worth calling about—but it's one of those times where *doing something small prevents something big.* Approach it together, calmly and quickly.

🗝 Takeaway

Bleeding after menopause doesn't automatically mean something serious, but it always deserves a look. Think of it as a flag on the play — not a foul, just a moment to pause, review, and make sure the next move is safe.

🩸 Section 15: Abnormal or Unexpected Bleeding Toolkit

"Flag on the Play: When to Call for Review"

Purpose:
Track any spotting, bleeding, or changes that happen during or after menopause. Bring this page to your next appointment — it helps your provider find patterns fast.

■ Bleeding Log

Date	Amount (Light/ Moderate/ Heavy)	Duration (Days)	Color (Bright/Dark)	Trigger (After Sex, Spontaneous, etc.)	Notes

---

■ Possible Contributing Factors

Factor	Present? (Y/N)	Notes
Hormone therapy changes		
New medications (blood thinners, supplements)		
Vaginal dryness or trauma		
Recent infection		
Exercise or intercourse		

■ Questions for My Provider

- ☐ Could this be from my uterus, cervix, or vagina?
- ☐ Do I need a pelvic ultrasound or biopsy?
- ☐ What's the thickness of my uterine lining?
- ☐ Should I stop or adjust my hormone therapy?
- ☐ How soon should I follow up?

Reflection Box

- ☐ My next GYN visit is scheduled for: ______________________________
- ☐ What I want to ask first: ______________________________

Partner Tip

If she tells you she's bleeding again, don't panic—but don't dismiss it either. Support her in calling the doctor promptly.

Section 16

Fast Breaks

Quick Answers for Common Questions

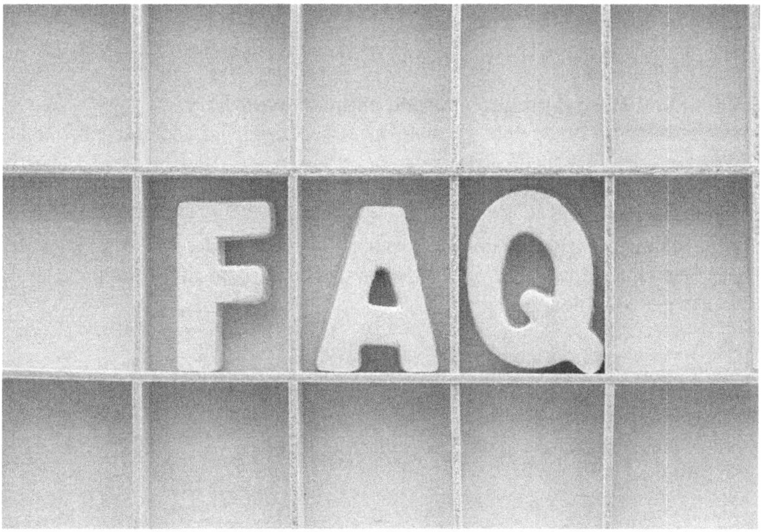

For Partners & Women (Read Together)

Every couple hits the point where you're both asking the same questions but not sure who to ask. These "fast breaks" give you the essentials — clear, short answers you can trust.

● The Basics

Q1. How long does menopause last?
Menopause itself is defined as 12 months without a period.
But the *transition* (perimenopause → postmenopause) can last **4–10 years.**

Q2. When does it usually start?
The average age in the U.S. is **51**, but symptoms often begin between **40–50.**

Q3. Can you still get pregnant during perimenopause?
Yes. Ovulation becomes unpredictable but still happens. Use contraception until you've had 12 months with no periods.

Q4. Is hormone therapy safe?
For most healthy women under 60 or within 10 years of menopause, **yes.** It's the most effective treatment for hot flashes and bone protection. Your provider will tailor it to your health profile.

Q5. Are there natural alternatives that work?
Yes — **some**. Exercise, plant-based foods, and certain supplements (like soy isoflavones or black cohosh) can help mild symptoms. Always check for medication interactions and discuss with your provider.

💬 Body Changes

Q6. Why do hot flashes happen?
Estrogen affects the brain's temperature control center. When levels drop, that thermostat "misfires," causing sudden heat waves.

Q7. Does everyone gain weight during menopause?
Not everyone — but metabolism slows, and fat redistributes toward the abdomen. Regular exercise and balanced meals help most.

Q8. Why does my sex drive feel different?
Estrogen loss, dryness, fatigue, and stress all play roles. Address physical causes (like dryness) and emotional ones (like stress or body image). Desire can return with comfort and connection.

Q9. Are mood swings normal?
Yes. Hormone shifts affect serotonin and dopamine, impacting mood and patience. If sadness or anxiety last more than two weeks, or you have any concerns about it, talk to your provider.

Q10. Is brain fog permanent?
No. It's usually temporary and improves as hormone levels stabilize, especially with sleep, exercise, and stress management.

🖤 Health & Prevention

Q11. Do I still need Pap smears and mammograms?
Yes — at least through age 65 for Pap tests and longer for mammograms. Menopause doesn't cancel screenings.

Q12. Should I see a cardiologist?
Ask your medical provider, Usually, if you have **high BP, high cholesterol, diabetes, or early menopause (<40)**, yes. Heart health becomes a bigger focus after estrogen declines.

Q13. Why do my joints ache now?
Estrogen helps reduce inflammation. Without it, stiffness and pain can increase. Movement, stretching, and adequate vitamin D help.

Q14. Can menopause affect my bladder?
Yes — tissues thin and weaken, leading to urgency or leakage. Pelvic floor exercises and vaginal estrogen can improve this.

Q15. Is it normal to feel sad or anxious?
Yes, but it's treatable. Counseling, mindfulness, and sometimes medication can make a big difference.

👩 Treatment & Care

Q16. What if I can't take hormone therapy?
You have options — SSRIs, SNRIs, gabapentin, etc, and lifestyle changes all help control hot flashes and mood.

Q17. How do I know if supplements are safe?
Always tell your provider what you're taking. Some herbs (like St. John's Wort) interfere with prescription meds. Look for **USP** or **NSF-certified** labels for quality.

Q18. When should I call my provider right away? Or call 911 if emergent.

- Any bleeding after menopause
- Chest pain, shortness of breath, or new swelling
- Severe or sudden headaches
- Leg pain or redness (possible blood clot)

Q19. Do I still need birth control after 50?
The guidelines say yes, until you've gone 12 months without a period. Some use low-dose IUDs or pills safely through perimenopause. Discuss with your provider.

Q20. Is there a "test" for menopause?
Blood tests for FSH and estradiol can confirm, but diagnosis is mostly based on symptoms and menstrual history.

💡 Bonus: Men Ask, Too

Q21. How can I help without making things worse?
Ask what she needs. Sometimes it's space; sometimes it's help. "I'm here if you need me" beats "You seem cranky."

Q22. Will sex ever feel normal again?
Yes, and often better. Comfort, confidence, and connection all return with the right care.

Q23. How long do these mood swings last?
They fade as hormones level out — but patience, humor, and rest speed recovery.

Q24. What's the best thing I can do?
Stay calm, informed, and available. Menopause is temporary; partnership is permanent.

🧩 Partner + Patient Perspective

Questions mean you're engaged — and that's a good sign. Curiosity builds confidence, and understanding replaces frustration.

🗝 Takeaway

Every couple's experience is different, but good information and teamwork make it easier. Don't be afraid to ask questions — that's how you stay ahead of the game.

Notes:

Notes:

Section 17

MythBusters

Clearing the Court for the Truth

Introduction

There's a lot of misinformation about menopause — from locker room jokes to social media "miracle cures." This chapter is here to call the fouls, clear the noise, and keep both partners on the same page.

Menopause isn't a disease. It's a normal, healthy transition that half the population goes through. But because it's rarely talked about openly, myths spread faster than facts.

Let's fix that — together.

● For Partners (Playbook Edition)

"Because no one gave you a rulebook."

Myth	The Reality
1. Menopause means she's done with intimacy.	False. Hormone changes may affect comfort or desire, but communication and treatment options make intimacy absolutely possible — often better than before.
2. Hot flashes are just mood swings.	Not even close. They're physical events triggered by estrogen loss that confuses the body's temperature control system.
3. Hormone therapy is dangerous for everyone.	False. For most healthy women under 60 or within 10 years of menopause, it's safe and effective under medical supervision.
4. If she's cranky, it's just hormones.	No — it's often exhaustion, heat, or frustration. Listen first; label later.

5. All women experience menopause the same way.	Not even close. Some breeze through it; others struggle for years. Comparing her to someone else just adds pressure.
6. This is her problem, not mine.	Wrong. Relationship changes, mood, intimacy, and routines all affect both partners. Support is part of the solution.
7. She's exaggerating her symptoms.	Not true. Studies show up to 80% of women have hot flashes, and half experience sleep or mood disruption.
8. Once it's over, everything goes back to normal.	Some symptoms fade, but heart, bone, and bladder health still need attention long-term.
9. Supplements are safer than prescription treatments.	"Natural" doesn't always mean safe. Always check with her provider before trying anything new.
10. Talking about menopause makes it worse.	The opposite. Open conversation lowers tension and improves connection.

💡 *Partner's takeaway:* The more you understand, the easier it is to support without guessing. You don't need to fix it — just show up informed.

❤ **For Women (Huddle Edition)** *"Because your body deserves facts, not fear."*

Myth	The Reality
1. Menopause starts the moment your period stops.	Not exactly. It's diagnosed after 12 months without a period. The transition (perimenopause) can start years earlier.
2. If my mom had it easy, I will too.	Genetics play a role, but lifestyle, stress, and health history matter just as much.
3. Weight gain is inevitable.	Metabolism slows, but regular exercise, strength training, and mindful eating can keep you healthy.
4. Hormone therapy causes cancer.	Outdated myth. Modern therapy is individualized and safe for most women; it's reviewed annually by your provider.
5. Hot flashes only happen at night.	They can happen anytime — during meetings, workouts, or sleep. Planning (fans, layers) helps manage them.
6. You can't build muscle after 50.	False. Resistance training builds strength and protects bones at any age.
7. Vaginal dryness is just something to live with.	Nope. Local estrogen, moisturizers, and lubricants work wonders.
8. You don't need gynecologic care after menopause.	Wrong. Screenings for bleeding, cancers, and prolapse remain important.
9. Brain fog means you're developing dementia.	No. Cognitive changes are temporary and tied to hormones and sleep — they improve over time.
10. Menopause means the end of vitality.	Absolutely not. It's the start of a new phase — one with wisdom, stability, and the freedom to focus on you.

💡 *Women's takeaway:* Menopause doesn't diminish you — it just redefines what strength looks like.

🧩 Partner + Patient Perspective

When both partners know the facts, misunderstandings disappear. The goal isn't to memorize medical details — it's to replace fear with teamwork and myths with mutual respect. Laughter counts as learning — myth-busting together keeps stress down and trust up.

🗝 Takeaway

Menopause isn't a mystery once you know the rules. Replace myths with facts, replace silence with humor, and keep your teamwork strong.

Notes:

Notes:

Section 18

Prevention & Long-Term Health

The Postseason Plan: Staying Strong for the Long Game

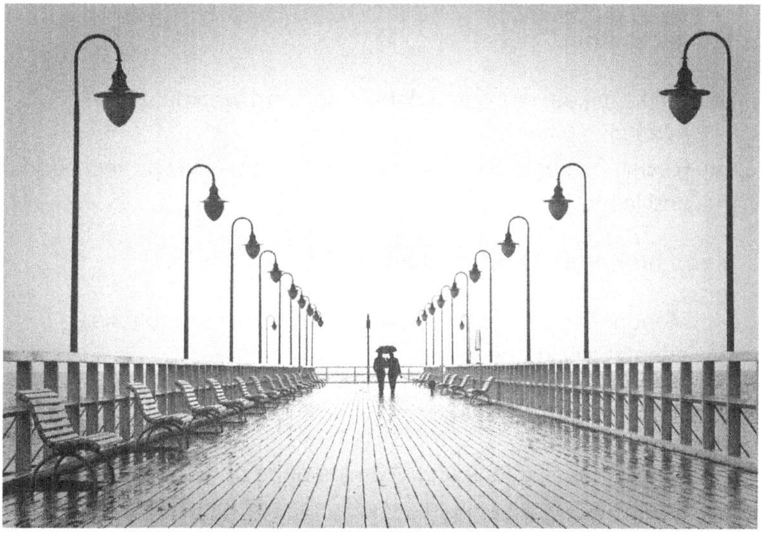

For Partners (Playbook)

Menopause isn't the end of the game — it's the **start of a new season.**
Now the focus shifts from symptom control to **staying healthy, active, and sharp** for decades to come.

Estrogen may have left the field, but good habits, strong relationships, and preventive care can take its place.
Here's how to keep your shared playbook working for both of you:

1. Encourage regular checkups.

- Primary care for blood pressure, cholesterol, and diabetes screening.
- GYN visits for pelvic health and cancer prevention.
- DEXA scans for bone strength.

2. Move together.

- Walks, hikes, or cycling double as heart workouts *and* relationship time.
- Resistance bands or light weights twice weekly protect bones and joints.

3. Keep humor and curiosity alive.

- Menopause can shift routines, intimacy, and emotions — adaptability keeps connection strong.

4. Plan the "health huddles."

- Review medications and vitamins once or twice a year.
- Keep track of screenings, vaccines, and labs together.

You're building stamina now — physically, emotionally, and relationally — for the long game ahead.

For Women (Huddle)

After menopause, prevention takes center stage. You've crossed the transition; now it's about **protecting your heart, bones, brain, and emotional health**.

Top Health Priorities After Menopause (per ACOG & ACC)

Focus	What to Do	Why It Matters
Heart Health	Control BP <120/80, eat heart-healthy, move 30 min/day	Heart disease is the #1 killer of women
Bone Health	Calcium 1,200 mg + Vit D 800 IU daily, DEXA every 2–5 yrs	Estrogen loss increases fracture risk
Cancer Prevention	Continue mammograms, colon screenings, Pap as advised	Early detection saves lives
Bladder & Pelvic Health	Do Kegels, manage weight, treat dryness early	Prevents incontinence, prolapse
Brain & Mental Health	Sleep, socialize, keep learning	Cognitive health stays sharp with engagement
Immunity	Flu, shingles, pneumonia, and COVID vaccines	Keeps defenses strong
Sexual Health	Maintain comfort with lubricants or local estrogen	Promotes circulation, intimacy, and tissue health

Distraction & Mindfulness Activities

Even prevention benefits from a calm mind and a little fun. These "distraction" activities keep anxiety down and resilience up:

- **Journaling:** Track gratitude or wins each day.
- **Puzzles & word games:** Keep cognition active.
- **Creative hobbies:** Painting, gardening, music, or crafting reduce stress hormones.
- **Stretch or yoga sessions:** Combine movement with mindfulness.
- **Volunteering or mentoring:** Purpose is protective — emotionally and physiologically.

💡 *Remember: stress management isn't indulgent — it's preventive medicine.*

Nutrition for Longevity

Menopause changes metabolism, but nutrition can keep you strong:

- Focus on *fiber, healthy fats, and lean protein.*
- Choose *whole foods over processed ones.*
- Hydrate — 8+ cups of water daily supports skin, joints, and bladder health.
- Limit added sugars; they accelerate inflammation and energy crashes.

Screening Schedule Cheat Sheet (per ACOG & USPSTF)

Screening	Frequency	Notes
Blood Pressure	Yearly	More often if elevated
Cholesterol & Glucose	Every 3–5 years (or sooner if abnormal)	Monitor cardiovascular risk
Mammogram	Every 1–2 years	Continue while healthy
Pap / HPV Test	Every 3–5 years until age 65	May stop if no abnormalities for 10 years
Colonoscopy	Every 10 years (or stool tests annually)	Choose method with your provider
DEXA (Bone Density)	Every 2–5 years	More often if osteopenia/osteoporosis
Dental / Eye Exams	Every 1–2 years	Oral and vision health affect aging
Skin Checks	Annually	Look for new or changing moles

🧩 Partner + Patient Perspective

The secret to long-term wellness isn't perfection — it's consistency.
When you plan health maintenance like you plan vacations or finances, you stay one step ahead.
Your partnership can be the accountability that keeps both of you thriving.

🗝 Takeaway

Menopause might change the pace, but it doesn't end the game. The "postseason" is about strength, stability, and joy — caring for your body and your bond so both can keep winning for decades to come.

Notes:

🖤 Section 18: Long-Term Health Toolkit

"The Postseason Plan: Staying Strong for the Long Game"

Purpose:
Track preventive care, vaccines, and long-range health goals for both partners.

🩺 Preventive Care Checklist

Screening / Test	Due Date	Done (✓)	Notes
Blood Pressure			
Cholesterol & Glucose			
Mammogram			
Colon Screening			
DEXA (Bone Density)			
Dental / Eye Exam			
Vaccines (Flu, Shingles, COVID, Tdap)			

🧘 Wellness Goals

Category	My Goal	Partner Goal	Notes
Exercise			
Nutrition			
Sleep			
Stress Relief			

💬 Reflection Box

- ☐ One habit I'll start this month: ______________________________

- ☐ One goal we'll share together: ______________________________

💡 Partner Tip

Plan wellness like you plan vacations — schedule it on purpose so it actually happens.

Section 19

Action Toolkit

Season Recap: What to Do Next

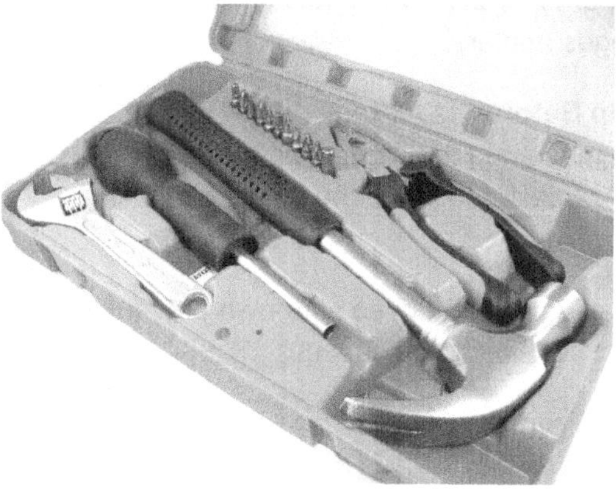

For Partners (Playbook)

The best teams don't just play hard — they review the game, make adjustments, and plan for the next season.
Menopause may have changed the playbook, but you've both learned the strategies to stay connected, healthy, and strong.

Here's your **Final Partner Playbook**:

1. Stay Curious.
Keep learning. Ask questions, listen without defensiveness, and keep humor alive.

2. Watch for Signals.
Encourage her to track how she feels — physically and emotionally. Subtle changes matter.

3. Offer Help Before It's Asked.
Whether it's managing the household, grocery runs, or bedtime routines, small gestures make the biggest impact.

4. Lead by Example.
Eat well, stay active, and keep your own preventive appointments. Shared effort equals shared success.

5. Celebrate Progress.
Menopause isn't a crisis — it's a phase. Mark the milestones: first symptom-free week, a good night's sleep, a successful doctor visit.

💡 *True partnership isn't about fixing; it's about showing up every day and choosing "us" again and again.*

For Women (Huddle)

You've done the hard part — navigating hormone shifts, body changes, and emotional waves.
Now it's time to build your **long-term game plan** for feeling healthy and confident.

Your Menopause Action Checklist *(Tear-out or fillable page in workbook)*

Focus Area	My Goal	Notes / Next Step
Symptoms	Track frequency and triggers	
Nutrition	Add more calcium, protein, and veggies	
Exercise	Walk 30 min/day, lift weights 2×/week	
Sleep	Create a nightly routine, limit screens	
Stress	Try meditation or deep breathing daily	
Heart Health	Get BP & cholesterol checked yearly	
Bone Health	Ask about DEXA scan	
Bladder & Pelvic Health	Do daily Kegels, treat dryness early	
Doctor Visits	Schedule annual physical & GYN visit	
Mental Health	Ask for help if mood changes persist	
Supplements / Meds	Review with provider annually	

Couple's Connection Plan *(A simple exercise to fill out together)*

1. One thing I'll try to do to support you better this month:
   ____
2. One thing I'd love more help with:
   ____
3. One shared goal for us this season (health, fun, or rest):
   ____
4. One way we'll relax together each week:
   ____

This turns small intentions into lifelong teamwork.

Red Flag Reminder (When to Call Your Provider or Seek immediate help)

- Any new **vaginal bleeding** after menopause
- **Chest pain, shortness of breath, or leg swelling**
- **Severe mood changes or depression**
- **Sudden vision changes or headaches**
- **Unexplained pain, weight loss, or fatigue**

Keep this list visible — it's not meant to scare you, just to empower you to act early.

🩺 Track Your Numbers (Tear-Out Page Option)

Metric	Goal Range	My Latest Result	Date
Blood Pressure	<120/80 mmHg		
Total Cholesterol	<200 mg/dL		
HDL (Good)	>50 mg/dL		
LDL (Bad)	<100 mg/dL		
Triglycerides	<150 mg/dL		
A1C (Blood Sugar)	<5.7%		
Weight / BMI			
Vitamin D Level	30–100 ng/mL		
DEXA (T-score)			

💡 *Tracking is power — not perfection. Even small improvements deserve celebration.*

Quick Recap Table: Your "Winning Season" Plan

Goal	How to Get There	Partner's Role
Manage symptoms	Use therapies + lifestyle changes	Encourage consistency
Stay healthy long-term	Exercise, nutrition, preventive care	Join in, model habits
Keep connection strong	Communicate, adapt intimacy	Listen, stay present
Maintain confidence	Self-care, humor, mindset	Offer affirmation
Prevent future issues	Regular screenings	Share planning & reminders

---

🧩 Partner + Patient Perspective

You've built a foundation for health and connection that can last decades.
The next step isn't about doing more — it's about living what you've learned.
Stay active, stay open, and keep choosing partnership over frustration.

🗝 Takeaway

Menopause isn't a finish line — it's a turning point.
The real victory is learning to care for your body and each other in new ways, with strength, humor, and love leading every play.

■ Section 19: Action Toolkit

"Season Recap: What to Do Next"

Purpose:
Use this final page as your all-in-one summary and tear-out reference.

■ My Next Steps

Goal	Deadline	Done (✓)
Schedule annual exam		
Review labs / BP		
Update supplements list		
Plan one stress-free activity per week		
Revisit Toolkits quarterly		

Couple's Connection Mini-Worksheet

1 Something I appreciate about you this month: ____________________
2 Something we did well as a team: ____________________
3 One thing I want to improve next month: ____________________
4 One fun goal for us to plan: ____________________

Keep in Mind

- Small changes compound over time.
- Communication is medicine.
- Every season has wins — track yours.

Partner Tip

End each week with a “five-minute huddle” — share a win, a challenge, and a laugh.

Notes:

Glossary

A

Adrenal Glands – Small glands on top of the kidneys that produce stress hormones (like cortisol) and small amounts of sex hormones after menopause.

Anxiety – Feelings of nervousness, restlessness, or fear that can increase during hormonal changes.

Atrophy (Vaginal or Urogenital) – Thinning and drying of vaginal and urinary tissues caused by low estrogen levels.

B

Balance Training – Exercises that improve stability and reduce fall risk, especially helpful for bone health.

Baseline – Your normal or starting point; often used when tracking blood pressure, weight, or lab results.

Bisphosphonates – Medications (like alendronate or risedronate) that slow bone loss and help prevent fractures.

Bladder Training – A technique to gradually retrain your bladder to hold urine longer and reduce urgency.

Body Mass Index (BMI) – A ratio of height and weight used to estimate healthy weight range.

Bone Density (DEXA) – A scan that measures bone strength and risk for osteoporosis.

C

Calcium – A mineral needed for strong bones, muscles, and nerves. Menopausal women need about 1,200 mg daily.
Cardiovascular Disease – Diseases that affect the heart and blood vessels; risk increases after menopause due to lower estrogen.
Cervix – The lower part of the uterus that opens into the vagina.
Cholesterol – A type of fat in the blood; includes “good” (HDL) and “bad” (LDL) types that affect heart health.
Clonidine – A non-hormonal medication that can help reduce hot flashes and lower blood pressure.
Cognitive Behavioral Therapy (CBT) – A form of talk therapy that helps change negative thought patterns; can help with mood and sleep during menopause.

D

DEXA Scan – A low-radiation test that measures bone density in the hips and spine.
DHEA (Dehydroepiandrosterone) – A hormone made by the adrenal glands; sometimes used in vaginal inserts to help dryness and tissue health.
Dietary Fiber – Plant-based carbohydrate that aids digestion, supports heart health, and reduces cholesterol.
Dopamine – A brain chemical that affects pleasure, motivation, and focus.
Dyspareunia – Medical term for pain during sex, often due to dryness or thinning tissue after menopause.

E

Endometrium – The inner lining of the uterus that builds up and sheds during menstrual cycles.

Endometrial Biopsy – A small sample of uterine tissue taken to check for abnormal cells or cancer.

Endorphins – "Feel-good" chemicals released during exercise that reduce pain and improve mood.

Estrogen – The primary female hormone made by the ovaries; supports bone, heart, and reproductive health.

Evening Primrose Oil – A plant supplement sometimes used for hot flashes; research shows limited benefit.

F

Fatigue – Ongoing tiredness or lack of energy; common during hormonal transitions.

Fezolinetant (Veozah) – A new FDA-approved, non-hormonal medication for moderate to severe hot flashes.

Fibroids – Noncancerous muscle growths in the uterus that can cause heavy bleeding or pelvic pressure.

Flaxseed – A source of plant estrogens and omega-3s; may mildly reduce hot flashes and improve heart health.

Follicle-Stimulating Hormone (FSH) – A hormone from the brain that increases when the ovaries stop releasing eggs.

G

Gabapentin – A medication originally for nerve pain and seizures, also used to treat hot flashes and night sweats.

Genitourinary Syndrome of Menopause (GSM) – Medical term for vaginal dryness, burning, urinary urgency, or discomfort due to low estrogen.

Gynecologist – A medical provider who specializes in women's reproductive health.

H

HDL (High-Density Lipoprotein) – The "good" cholesterol that protects heart health.

Hormone Replacement Therapy (HRT or HT) – Treatment that replaces estrogen (and sometimes progesterone) to relieve symptoms and protect bones.

Hot Flashes – Sudden feelings of warmth, sweating, or flushing caused by changes in estrogen levels.

Hydration – Adequate water intake; supports skin, bladder, and body temperature regulation.

Hyperplasia (Endometrial) – Thickening of the uterine lining that sometimes causes abnormal bleeding.

I

Insomnia – Trouble falling or staying asleep, often linked to hot flashes or anxiety.

Isoflavones – Plant-based compounds (found in soy) that act like mild estrogens.

Inflammation – The body's response to stress or injury; can worsen joint pain or fatigue during menopause.

J

Joint Pain – Common after menopause due to inflammation and reduced estrogen support for cartilage.
Journaling – Writing thoughts or feelings daily to reduce stress and improve mood.

K

Kegel Exercises – Pelvic floor muscle exercises that strengthen bladder and vaginal support.
Kidneys – Organs that filter waste from blood and help control fluid balance and blood pressure.

L

LDL (Low-Density Lipoprotein) – The "bad" cholesterol that can build up in arteries and increase heart risk.
Libido – Sexual desire; often influenced by hormones, mood, and physical comfort.
Lifestyle Medicine – Using healthy habits (diet, exercise, sleep, stress control) as part of medical care.

M

Menopause – The stage reached after 12 consecutive months without a menstrual period, marking the end of fertility.
Metabolism – The rate at which your body converts food into energy; often slows with age and low estrogen.
Mindfulness – Awareness and acceptance of the present moment, used to reduce stress and anxiety.
Mood Swings – Sudden emotional changes due to fluctuating estrogen and serotonin.

N

Night Sweats – Hot flashes that happen during sleep, often soaking clothing or bedding.

Non-Hormonal Therapy – Treatments that relieve menopause symptoms without estrogen or progesterone (like SSRIs or gabapentin).

Nutrition – The balance of foods and nutrients needed for health, energy, and disease prevention.

O

Oophorectomy – Surgical removal of the ovaries; causes immediate menopause.

Osteopenia – Lower-than-normal bone density, a precursor to osteoporosis.

Osteoporosis – A disease that weakens bones, making them more likely to break.

Ospemifene – A non-hormonal medication that improves vaginal comfort and elasticity.

Ovulation – Release of an egg from the ovary; becomes irregular during perimenopause and stops at menopause.

P

Pap Smear (Pap Test) – Screening for cervical cancer by collecting cells from the cervix.

Pelvic Floor – Group of muscles that support the bladder, uterus, and rectum.

Perimenopause – The transition phase before menopause when hormones fluctuate and symptoms begin.

Phytoestrogens – Natural plant compounds that act like mild estrogens in the body.

Progesterone – A hormone that balances estrogen and regulates menstrual cycles.

Prolapse – When pelvic organs drop from their normal position due to weak support tissues.

Q

Quality of Life – Overall sense of well-being; includes physical, mental, and emotional health.

R

Raloxifene – A medication that acts like estrogen on bones but not breast or uterus tissue.

Resistance Training – Strength exercises using weights or bands to build muscle and bone.

Risk Factors – Habits or conditions that increase chances of disease (like smoking, obesity, or family history).

S

Serotonin – A brain chemical that helps regulate mood, sleep, and emotion; decreases with estrogen loss.
Sleep Hygiene – Habits that improve sleep, like consistent bedtime and screen limits.
Soy – A plant rich in isoflavones, which may help mild menopause symptoms.
Statins – Medications that lower cholesterol to protect heart health.
Stress Incontinence – Leaking urine when sneezing, coughing, or laughing due to weak pelvic muscles.

T

Testosterone – A hormone made in small amounts by women; supports libido and energy.
Thyroid – A gland in the neck that controls metabolism and energy levels.
Triglycerides – Blood fats that increase with poor diet or inactivity; linked to heart disease.
TSH (Thyroid-Stimulating Hormone) – A blood test that checks thyroid function.

U

Urge Incontinence – Sudden need to urinate, sometimes leading to leakage.
Urethra – The tube that carries urine out of the body.
Uterus – The womb; where periods originate and pregnancy develops.

V

Vaginal Estrogen – Localized estrogen therapy that restores tissue comfort without raising body-wide hormone levels.
Vaginal Moisturizer – OTC product that hydrates tissue for long-term comfort.
Venlafaxine (Effexor) – An antidepressant that can also relieve hot flashes.
Vitamin D – Helps the body absorb calcium and maintain bone health.

W

Weight-Bearing Exercise – Activities like walking or dancing that use body weight to strengthen bones.
Wellness – A state of balance between body, mind, and environment — not just absence of disease.

X

X-Ray (DEXA-related) – Imaging test using small doses of radiation to measure bone mineral density.

Y

Yoga – Mind-body practice combining stretching, breathing, and relaxation; proven to reduce stress and hot flashes.

Z

Zinc – A mineral that supports immune function and wound healing; found in nuts, meat, and legumes.

Appendix E – Trusted Resources & National Organizations

(Cited from academic societies and national health agencies)

Menopause & Women's Health:

American College of Obstetricians and Gynecologists (ACOG)
www.acog.org → *Patient FAQs and Practice Bulletins on Menopause, Hormone Therapy, and Preventive Care*

The North American Menopause Society (NAMS)
www.menopause.org → *Menopause Basics, Position Statements, and Clinician Finder*

U.S. Department of Health & Human Services Office on Women's Health (OWH)
www.womenshealth.gov/menopause → *Educational Handouts and Lifestyle Tips*

National Institute on Aging (NIA), NIH
www.nia.nih.gov/health/menopause → *Evidence-based articles for midlife women*

Bone & Musculoskeletal Health:

Bone Health & Osteoporosis Foundation (BHOF, formerly NOF)
www.bonehealthandosteoporosis.org → *Calcium/Vitamin D guidelines and DEXA resources*

American College of Rheumatology (ACR)
www.rheumatology.org → *Clinical info on osteoporosis and joint care*

Heart & Metabolic Health:

American Heart Association (AHA)
www.heart.org → *Go Red for Women campaign and heart-risk tools*

American College of Cardiology (ACC)
www.acc.org → *Guidelines on women's cardiovascular risk and prevention*

Pelvic Floor & Sexual Health:

International Society for the Study of Women's Sexual Health (ISSWSH)
www.isswsh.org → *Educational statements on sexual function and GSM care*

American Urogynecologic Society (AUGS)
www.augs.org → *Resources on incontinence and pelvic floor therapy*

Mental & Emotional Wellness:

National Alliance on Mental Illness (NAMI)

www.nami.org → *Hotlines and local support groups*

American Psychological Association (APA)
www.apa.org/topics/menopause → *Mind-body strategies and therapy options*

Cancer & Surgical Recovery:

American Cancer Society (ACS)
www.cancer.org → *Guidelines on hormone-sensitive cancers and survivorship care*

National Comprehensive Cancer Network (NCCN)
www.nccn.org/patients → *Evidence-based patient guidelines*

Lifestyle & Nutrition:

Academy of Nutrition and Dietetics (AND)
www.eatright.org → *Menopause-specific nutrition articles and meal planning*

Centers for Disease Control and Prevention (CDC)
www.cdc.gov/women → *Preventive screening and vaccine schedules*

Hotlines & Support:

988 Suicide & Crisis Lifeline – Call 988 (24/7, free, confidential)

NAMI Helpline: 1-800-950-6264 (M-F 10 AM–10 PM ET)

OWH Women's Health Information Center: 1-800-994-9662 (M-F 9 AM–6 PM ET)

Citation Note

All medical definitions and statistics throughout this book are based on publications from the **American College of Obstetricians and Gynecologists (ACOG)**, **The North American Menopause Society (NAMS)**, **UpToDate**, **American College of Cardiology (ACC)**, **Bone Health & Osteoporosis Foundation (BHOF)**, and **U.S. Department of Health & Human Services Office on Women's Health (OWH)** as of 2025.

Quick Index

About the Author

Stacie the PA

Duke residency-trained Physician Assistant with over 20 years of clinical experience, Stacie the PA is known for turning complex medical topics into clear, compassionate, and practical guides that empower patients to take charge of their health.

Through her **Medical Things Explained** company and her ongoing work in the field of medicine, Stacie creates resources designed for real people — patients, partners, and providers — who want trustworthy, plain-language explanations backed by science.

When she's not writing, she's teaching, mentoring new providers, or enjoying time with her husband and their dachshunds.

📚 More Helpful Books by Stacie the PA

Clear, compassionate, and practical guides written by a medical provider who cares.

💧 **Kidney Stones 101**
A clear guide to causes, treatments, and prevention strategies.

💓 **Hypertension 101**
Understand high blood pressure and how to manage it — simply.

🦵 **Knee Pain 101**
From anatomy to treatment options, a complete patient reference.

🦴 **Hip Pain 101**
Everything you need to know about hip pain, diagnosis, and care.

💪 **Shoulder Pain 101**
An easy-to-follow guide to common shoulder problems and solutions.

🧠 **Neck Pain 101**
An easy-to-follow guide to spine-related neck pain, diagnosis, and treatment options.

🫁 **Pneumonia 101**
Learn the basics of prevention, symptoms, and recovery.

🔥 **Gout 101**
Practical answers about causes, flares, and long-term care.

🦠 **Diverticulosis 101**
Understand symptoms, triggers, and treatment of this common digestive condition.

🎗 **Breast Cancer 101: A Patient's Complete Guide to Symptoms, Treatments, and Prevention**
A compassionate, evidence-based guide for patients, survivors,

and caregivers — covering everything from diagnosis to recovery and long-term wellness.

🎗 **Cáncer de Mama 101: Guía Completa para Pacientes**
The Spanish-language edition of *Breast Cancer 101* — designed to serve North American Spanish-speaking patients and families with the same supportive, educational approach.

🌟 **Coming Soon: Menopause 101 in Spanish, and Back Pain 101:** A complete guide to understanding, treating, and preventing back pain.

🌐 Stay Connected

Follow for updates, educational content, and patient-friendly health tips:

Website: https://staciethepa.com/
Amazon Author Page: Stacie the PA on Amazon
Social: @StacieThePA

💡 Affiliate Note

Some of the links on my website or author page may be affiliate links. This means I may earn a small commission if you purchase through them — at no additional cost to you.
These proceeds help fund the creation of more patient-education books, toolkits, and free online resources.

Thank you for your support!

Francis Galton on Mars

The 'Discontinuous Variation' Notebook

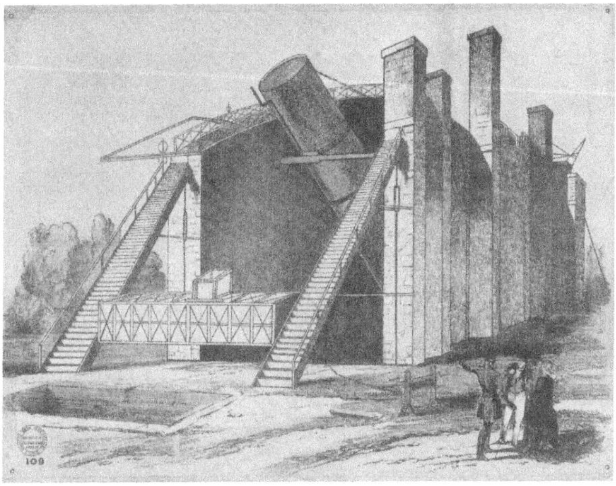

Edited by Gavan Tredoux

galton.org

ISBN: 978-1-963225-13-6
Not for sale in the United Kingdom.

Francis Galton: a Lifetime of Exploration.

1. *Francis Galton's Nature and Nurture:* 1822–1865.
2. *Francis Galton's Genius:* 1865–1911.

Supplements:

1. *Sir Francis Sacheverel Darwin:* Charles Darwin's Adventurous Uncle.
2. *Francis Galton at Cambridge:* Letters and Diaries, 1840–1844.
3. *The Diary of Charles John Andersson:* 1850–1851.
4. *Francis Galton on Mars:* the Discontinuous Variation Notebook.
5. *Francis Galton and Alphonse de Candolle:* Notes and Correspondence.
6. *Francis Galton and Alfred Binet:* Correspondence.
7. *Francis Galton:* Selected Papers, Notebooks and Diaries.

Contents

Chapter 1

Preface

Among the Galton papers, housed in the Special Collections Department of University College London, many notebooks survive, recording his explorations of things that amused him or took his fancy. Much of this material never saw print. The pages teem with ideas, often skipping around without warning.[1]

One of these notebooks is titled 'Discontinuous Variation: 1896-7'. The first page leads with 'Clear mind from cant' and contains ruminations about moral philosophy and religion. 'Ideals may well be elusive'. Several of the subsequent pages reflect the title, dealing with the ways in which change in a continuous characteristic can eventually produce a discontinuity, so that a different class is called for. By the twenty-second page, the subject has jumped to free

[1] For an overview of Galton's career and legacy, see `http://galton.org`.

will, a recurring theme for Galton, prompted by his researches into heredity. Three pages later, the subject switches abruptly to an encoding scheme for representing mathematical operations. Seventeen pages of rough notes follow, in which the scope of the encoding expands to include instructions for reproducing pictures. Encoding of pictures forms a link to 'Discontinuous variation', since at a certain point a series of dots is perceived as a line. On the forty-second page of the notebook, Galton lays out the skeleton of a story involving Mars, sun signals flashed from Earth, and eugenics among intelligent Martians, who are said to be descended from Ants by natural and artificial selection. It is only on page 79—three from the end, dated May 1897—that the subject switches once again, to the mathematics of descent.

The semi-comical 'short story' that lies between God and the beginnings of mathematical genetics was born in 1892, only to be more or less abandoned by 1896, when it was suddenly taken up again. Then, some ideas from it were transformed for use in 'Intelligible Signals between neighbouring stars', which was published in 1896 in the *Fortnightly Review*, alongside Olive Schreiner and Edward Dicey on the Jameson Raid, E. Ray Lankester on 'The Present Evolution of Man' and Alfred Russel Wallace on the Swiss Gorge of the Aar. But the published version left out many of the best bits.[2]

Intriguingly, sections of the unpublished story anticipate Galton's lost comic dystopia, *Kantsaywhere*, where procreation depends on rigorous eugenic examinations. Quite possibly he thought that the Victorian reading public was not ready for this in 1896—the editors of the *Fortnightly* accepted his story as it was submitted to them, so they were not to blame. Aside from leaving out the eugenic details and humorous Martian anthropology—or rather, entomology—the focus of the action was shifted 180°. In the unpublished original, it is the Martians who receive the glimmering signals, and they dictate the point of view of the narrative. In the parts that survived selection for the *Fortnightly*, it is Earth that receives the signals, and so a lot of diverting humour is lost.

Astronomy was more than a passing interest for Galton. On the board the *Dalhousie* to South-West Africa, in April of 1850, he had learned the use of the sextant and how to take latitudes. He fell in love with the instrument and the activity itself. In the field, taking readings occupied a great deal of his time, and the record of his trip was remarkable for its accurate surveying and painstaking observations, with multiple levels of redundancy to allow for error correction. Later, in successive editions of his *vade*

[2] Galton 1896a. See Appendix A, p. 89.

mecum for explorers, *The Art of Travel*, Galton took care to cover navigation by the stars. 'It requires very great practice to steer well by stars, for, on an average, they change their bearings even faster than they change their altitudes. In tropical countries the zodiacal stars, as Orion and Antares, give excellent east and west points. The Great Bear is useful, when the North Pole cannot be seen, for you may calculate by the eye whereabouts it would be in the heavens when its "pointers" were vertical, or due north; and the Southern Cross is available in precisely the same way.'[3]

On his return to England from Africa, fêted by the Royal Geographical Society, Galton often dined with Lord Rosse, an old friend of his (deceased) father Samuel Tertius, who had abiding interests in amateur astronomy. Rosse had built the world's largest telescope, the six-foot 'Leviathan', at his estate in Parsonstown Ireland. Despite his unpromising location, Rosse discovered what were later recognized to be remote galaxies using it. The intricate engineering problems solved by the versatile peer surely intrigued Galton.

Galton had also accompanied George Airy's expedition to Spain in 1860, to witness that year's solar eclipse from the clear-skied valley of the Ebro. The

3 Galton 1856b, 127.

large and delicate thermometer he had taken with to record changes in temperature—an instrument designed by J. W. F. Herschel—had been broken in transit, freeing him to make his own observations by eye. He was one of the first to notice the curvature effect at the perimeter of the sun, and the watercolour he painted of the view was reprinted more than once, though only in monochrome.[4] Whenever he had the opportunity to record the paths of meteors, he was suitably equipped with a compact travelling altazimuth, which he seems to have carried around with him on the off chance that it would prove useful.[5] But these interests, unlike his ethnological and geographical concerns, did not rise to an active role in bodies like the Astronomical Society.

The use of sunlight for signals was familiar to Galton from a much earlier date. In the Lake District in 1841, he noticed the (cumbersome) heliostats then in use. 'I found a small encampment of ordnance surveyors with theodolite and heliostat. Their immediate object was to obtain by direct observation the bearing of Snowdon, ninety-six miles off (as I think they said), to form the side of one of their principal triangles. A corresponding station was set up on the

4 Galton 1861, 1879. For full details on this expedition, see Tredoux 2023.
5 Galton 1866.

top of Snowdon, whence after many days' waiting in vain the long-wished-for star of light reflected from the sun by the mirror on Snowdon, became faintly but clearly visible through the telescope at Scawfell.'[6] C. F. Gauss invented one of the early heliographs from that period.

In 1856, in a letter to the *Times*, 'Signals Available to Men who are Adrift on Wrecks at Sea', Galton suggested that shipwrecked sailors might carry a mirror to attract the attention of passing ships—notoriously blind to their presence. He carefully described how the challenging task of aiming the flash might be accomplished even in a lifeboat, by scratching a small hole in the backing of the mirror to look through: 'a man sitting low down in the stern could direct the glitter of his looking glass by watching its play upon the bows of the boat at the moment when he could just catch sight of the ship over them. If a looking glass be used without first cutting a hole in its back in the way I have mentioned it is necessary to hold it close up under the eye, and to make more careful allowance for the height of the eye above it than a person who has not had a good deal of practice is likely to succeed in accomplishing.'[7]

6 Galton 1908, 61.

7 Galton 1856a. See Appendix B, p. 115. Galton had taken in the Naval Review on the 23rd.

Within two years, Galton had gone much further and invented a portable 'pocket' heliostat, which included a simple and reliable mechanism for visually aiming the instrument, through mirrors, which showed the user a 'mock sun' where the light would fall. Successive editions of Galton's *Art of Travel* described the instrument and the general problem of signalling in the wild.[8]

The invention eventually proved to be a success, after some refinements. It was initially manufactured by Troughton and Sims, then by other makers like John Dennett Potter, and widely used in practice by the Hydrographic Office. Galton carried one himself on his travels, and enjoyed whiling away the hours practicing its use in the mountains, and calibrating its visibility under different conditions. William Wharton was still recommending it at the turn of the century. 'A better instrument is the excellent and convenient Galton's Sun Signal, now also supplied. This is fitted with a telescope, by looking through which and adjusting the mirror, a dim image of the sun is seen covering the object required to flash to. Nothing can be better adapted to the purposes of the nautical surveyor's work than this (when he is once accustomed to it, as at first it is a little awkward to manage), and when obtainable they should always be

[8] Galton 1855, 1856b, 1858, 1860, 1867, 1872.

used.'[9] In 1911, the *Encyclopedia Britannica* noted that Galton's sun signal was the most convenient of the heliostats used for surveying. The instrument was certainly widely used for coastal surveys.[10]

Mars had drawn Galton's attention as early as 1892, when he wrote a letter to the *Times* ruminating on the possibility of flashing sun signals at the planet, in the hope that Martians with telescopes might see the glimmering.[11] The planet was much in the news at that time. It was set to be unusually close to Earth that year, and there had in the past been reports from Giovanni Schiaparelli in Italy, and Camille Flammarion in France, among others, that canal-like structures were clearly visible on its surface.[12] Various observers even claimed that lights had been seen twinkling on the planet.

> SUN SIGNALS TO MARS.
> TO THE EDITOR OF THE TIMES.
>
> Sir,—Two facts appear in the papers—the one that an old French lady bequeathed

[9] William Wharton *Hydrographical Surveying* (1898), 35.

[10] *Encyclopedia Britannica*, Vol. 26, 'Surveying', 154. See also the *Official Catalogue and Guide* for the Naval Exhibition (1891).

[11] Galton 1892.

[12] Percival Lowell pursued this idea vigorously in the United States from 1893/4 onward.

a considerable sum for attempts to communicate with the planets, which has been perhaps rashly rejected; the other is that the planet Mars is now so near as that the exceptionally large magnifying power usable at the Lick Observatory[13] brings it optically to within 50,000 miles. To these I will add a third fact, derived from my own experiences in sun-signalling many years ago by a method described in the "Art of Travel." It then appeared that a reflected beam of sunlight sent through a hole in a plate in front of the mirror was just distinctly visible as a faint glint at a distance of ten miles when the hole was a square of one-tenth of an inch in the side. The amount of fog and haze that beam of light would traverse between us and Mars when the planet was high above our horizon could not exceed that along a terrestrial base of ten miles; consequently the same proportion between the size of mirror and the distance would still hold true. It follows that the flash from many mirrors simultaneously, whose aggregate width was 15 yards, and whose aggregate length (to allow for slope) was, say, 25 yards, would be visi-

[13] In California, near San Jose.

ble in Mars if seen through a telescope such as that at the Lick Observatory. With funds and good will, there seems no insuperable difficulty in flashing from a very much larger surface than the above, and sending signals that the inhabitants of Mars, if they have eyes, wits, and fairly good telescopes, would speculate on and wish to answer. One, two, three, might be slowly flashed over and over again from us to them, and possibly in some years, to allow time for speculation in Mars to bear practical fruit, one, two, three, might come back in response. Dr. Whewell, if I recollect right, wrote a paper on the possibility of coming to an understanding with lunar inhabitants, if there were any. He would begin from the mathematical side.

The practical difficulty is by no means insuperable of enabling many independent observers (who need not be near together) to direct their flashes aright. If mirrors could be mounted without much cost as heliostats (and perhaps they can be) it would be easy enough to do this. My own method is not practicable, at least without considerable addition and modifications, as it requires the object to be visible towards which the flash is directed, but Mars is not visible to the naked eye at day.

FRANCIS GALTON.

An anonymous writer in the *Sheffield Independent* demurred. 'For my part, I confess, a gentlemen in Mars might signal to me from morning to night without my having the least idea not only of what he wanted, but that he was signalling.' And, slyly, that although canals were detected on Mars by an American observer, the fact that boats were not seen on them may have been due to the destructive effects of competition from the railways.[14] Likewise the killjoy *Spectator* insisted that mankind had no idea whether 'Martials' existed in the first place, whether they could see or what they might look like, and doubted whether any common language could be found to allow one party to understand the other.[15]

On September the 8th, Norman Lockyer took up the idea in *Nature*, repeating the contents of the *Times* letter, and contrasting it to a proposal put forward by the Rev. Hugh Reginald Haweis, who suggested using a giant battery of London's electric street lights in concert to send signals. The drawback of using sunlight would be that Mars would see the earth lit by

[14] *Sheffield Independent*, Wednesday 24 August 1892, 4.
[15] See Appendix D, p. 121.

the sun, without the desired contrast. Electric lights seemed more promising to Lockyer.[16]

Galton 'dashed off' a response to the discussion his letter had sparked off. A draft survives in the Galton Papers at University College London, and for once really is entirely on the back of an envelope.[17] It is prefaced by a note added by Galton much later. 'Interplanetary language. Draft of a letter to *Spectator*, they sent me a proof but did not eventually publish it'. However, the contents show that this is an error—see the reference to 'yours' below. The letter was probably intended for Galton's old sub-editor from his *Reader* days, Norman Lockyer, and his journal *Nature*.

> Being at some distance from London, I have of late seen & shall see few newspapers, but have noticed in the *Spectator* of last week a reference to previous remarks of yours on the narrowness of the possible communication with Mars, supposing free communication by flashes to be feasible. It would seem that you limited it to the response of the 3 flashes suggested by myself as a mere illustration in a letter to the

16 J. Norman Lockyer, 'The Opposition of Mars', *Nature* 46, 08 September 1892, 443–448.

17 GALTON/2/10/9.

Times. But very much more than this would be possible, under the supposed circumstances. It is an interesting subject & worth writing a few lines about. We could literally probe their knowledge of algebra & the civil service. [I discuss what Whewell proposed as unsuitable to the easy] [... geometrical problems] Examiners could examine them, if both parties were pleased to take the trouble of acting as examiners and examinees. We could teach advanced mathematics to them, and learn from them. To simplify the explanation of how this [is done] let a dot · mean a flash followed by an interval, and let any word in brackets signify some appropriate combination of dot and dash symbols that would always be used by us to signify the sense of word or phrase, but which is supposed as yet to be unknown to the people in Mars. When it is known let it be written in italics.

First experiment (a) Flash (plus) Flash (equal) Flash Flash. (b) Flash (plus) Flash Flash (equal) Flash Flash Flash. (c) Flash Flash (plus) Flash (equal) Flash Flash Flash

Anybody in Mars with the smallest algebraic knowledge would understand that (plus) meant Plus, and (equal) meant equal, & would respond by analogous signals such as Flash Flash (plus) Flash (equal) Flash Flash Flash &c. To this we should send back (right)

By an analogous fashion (minus) would be understood & after a while (wrong).

So we have already got plus minus equal [...] right wrong

Next might come fl: fl: (multiplied into) fl: fl: (equal) fl: fl: fl: fl: then ... (divided by) ... (equal) .... Then square & cube; square root & cube roots. The knowledge of the symbol for equal would enable (symbolic) names of the numbers to be communicated thus dot dot = dot dot dot − dot = dot plus dot = (two) & so on. Next the symbol for (raised to the power of) 2 = 4.

Next try binomial expansions $(2+1)^2 =$ 4+4+1 $(2+2)^2 = 4 + 8 + 4$ $(2+1)^2$ $(2+2)^3$ &c. & finally when that was quite clearly taken $((a)+(b))^{(n)}$. Every one of which unknown symbols after so much preparatory leading, the Martials would make out. Sine & cosine &c. would be conveyed by their algebraical expressions and by running algebraic expressions side by side with their

> geometric equivalents, a considerable number of useful words would be in time determined: circle, line, intersection, angle, perpendicular, square, rectangle &c. Then the formulae for gravity & the numerical values that we know, for that at the surface of Mars to which they w^{d} respond to. Give that at the surface of Venus [...][18]

In January of 1893, Galton developed his information encoding and transmission ideas in the second part of a public lecture at the Royal Institution, on the 'Just Perceptible Difference'.[19] Even though it was held on a Friday evening, it was well-attended. The cyclostyle was then in wide use for creating copies of documents using a stencil, on the principle that discrete dots of ink placed sufficiently close to each other appeared to be continuous. Experimentally it had been found that at the reading distance of one foot, 300 dots per inch (an angle of one minute of a degree) appeared to be continuous. However the cyclostyle economised at a 'good enough' 140 dots per inch.

Galton described a scheme for encoding pictures using 26 alphabetical characters. Letters a to p gave compass directions from reference points, starting from north, clockwise. Z is used to signal 'end' (of the

[18] Cut off here.
[19] Galton 1893.

segment from the current reference point). To allow movement with no corresponding marks, to capture isolated parts of a figure, R and S could be used to delimit the invisible moves. The remainder of the letters were reserved for establishing and then moving the reference points. In this way a sequence of letters, grouped for convenience into words of at most 5 letters, could be used to encode a picture, transmit it by telegraph, and reconstruct it on the other side. A fragment of a picture might look like the following, which draws the eye of a Greek portrait of a girl (see Figure 1.5, p. 25). The encoding starts from the reference point U on the brow, and makes the sequence of invisible moves between R and S, before outlining the eye from the new reference point V:

> URkkk kklll mSVap pomnn mralmm mhnlm llmZZ VnTnn mnmmm mmmlm mmnZZ Tjjjj jjkkc chmm mnnn onoo

A second encoding scheme was also described, using a numerical grid of coordinate moves, centered at (4, 4), or 44. This allowed for finer control, with 63 moves from each successive dot, up to 3 spaces at a time—but at the expense of a longer encoding (see Figure 1.6, p. 26). This come closest to what modern readers will recognize as a digital encoding of an analogue picture, e.g. 21, 31, 62, ...

In private, Galton worked out the preliminary details of Martian signalling, but put the work aside when general enthusiasm for the remote planet temporarily faded. Nevertheless, the reading public had been following the conversation. In 1895, in the short story 'Message from Mars', a professor of mechanical engineering at Bristol University again took up the idea of communications with Mars by means of light. Few technical details were given, though the possibility of communicating shapes and numbers by spectra was mentioned.[20]

In the following year, 1896, Galton was taking one of his annual continental soaking cures, this time in Germany at the Wildbad spa. On the 19th of June he had suffered another attack of 'gastric catarrh' (most likely what is now called gastritis), and was packed off to the spa on July the 10th by the family physician of long-standing, Dr. Dobrée Chepmell.[21] Finding himself with time to spare, as the rain had set in generally, for weeks, he picked up the notebook again. Increasing deafness meant that other distractions were limited anyway. Internal evidence from the notebook implies that he was working on the Martian

[20] John Munro (1849–1930), 'Message from Mars' in *Cassell's Family Magazine*, 1895, 292.

[21] For Chepmell, Dr. Isaac Dobrée, see page 157.

theme again by July the 29th of 1896, and that all the text in the notebook related to this dates from that period.

Now Galton placed his bootstrapping information encoding scheme within a science-fiction vehicle, letting his imagination loose. The residents of Mars, who it so happens are the descendants of Ant-like creatures, with faces like diving helmets, are startled to see flashes from Earth. Newspaper controversy ensues in the *Bellona Gazette.* Speculation about the nature of the earthlings runs rife. An expensive telescope is constructed despite budget hardliners. The messages are decoded using the bootstrapping principle, starting from elementary arithmetic. As an introduction to these events, the narrator describes the morphology of the Martians, and their eugenic practices, whereby natural selection has been enhanced.

According to Louisa's yearly record, the Galtons were back in England by September the 7th—by way of Oberstdorf, Davos, Zurich, Freiburg, Strassburg & Rheims—so Frank had about a month and half all told to work on the story. Back in England, or perhaps even earlier on the continent, after Wildbad, Galton rewrote and edited the piece down to the form it took in the *Fortnightly,* where it appeared in the November issue. Correspondence with the editor, W. L. Courtney, shows that the piece must have been submitted in September at the latest, as it was accepted by October the 2nd. The manuscript of the neutered version, with its inversion of the roles of Martians and 'earthlings', has not survived.

But before Galton's piece was even published, the newspapers managed to garble the details, drawing the following testy complaint.

> SIGNALLING FROM MARS.[22]
>
> TO THE EDITOR OF THE STANDARD.
>
> Sir,—In the Article in *The Standard* on my paper in the forthcoming "Fortnightly," you say: "The result in his imaginary case was that, in the course of about three and a-half years, the terrestrial astronomers had been taught a code ..."[23] I said and showed that three and a-half hours would suffice, which makes much difference in the interest of what I endeavoured to explain. I am, Sir, your obedient servant, FRANCIS GALTON. 42, Rutland-gate, S.W., October 28.

Still, the advance notice in the *Evening Standard* shows how seriously the thoughts of Galton, as a leading member of the Royal Society and other bodies, were taken even on topics as remote from his usual remit as interplanetary communication.

[22] Galton 1896b.

[23] See *London Evening Standard*, Wednesday 28 October 1896, 5.

The *Globe*, the *Illustrated London News* and the Guernsey *Star* were enthusiastic about Galton's proposition and flights of fancy.[24] For skepticism one had to go further north, to Sheffield, where the *Independent* was not impressed. 'To attempt to communicate with Mars would leave the combined millionaires of the world out at elbows, and might in the end be as much use as an oration to an ash-heap. On the whole, in spite of learned articles in half-crown reviews, it is wiser to wait until our planetary neighbours begin.'[25]

The Mars notes and all their elaborations show the inventiveness, the broad reach and the all too often neglected comic side of Galton, a man who could turn his attention to almost any subject and get interesting results. Previously only a few fragments of the text have appeared in Derek Forrest's biography of Galton.[26] The full text is reproduced here for the first time, reconstructed from Galton's very rough form, along with the *Fortnightly Review* version and other interesting pages from the notebook, on subjects such as discontinuous variation, classification, religion and moral philosophy.

Uncertain constructions appear in square brackets, e.g. [doubtful], whereas occasionally illegible sec-

[24] Wednesday 28 October 1896, 1; Saturday 12 December 1896, 19, 20; Saturday 31 October 1896.

[25] *Sheffield Independent*, Wednesday 04 November 1896, 4.

[26] Forrest 1974, 237–240.

tions appear in ellipsis, e.g. [...]. Illustrations in the text are taken from the images of the notebook to be found in the Galton Papers in the Wellcome Collection, following the terms of the 'Creative Commons Attribution 4.0 International licence' appearing there.[27]

Gavan Tredoux
November 2018.

[27] See `https://wellcomelibrary.org`.

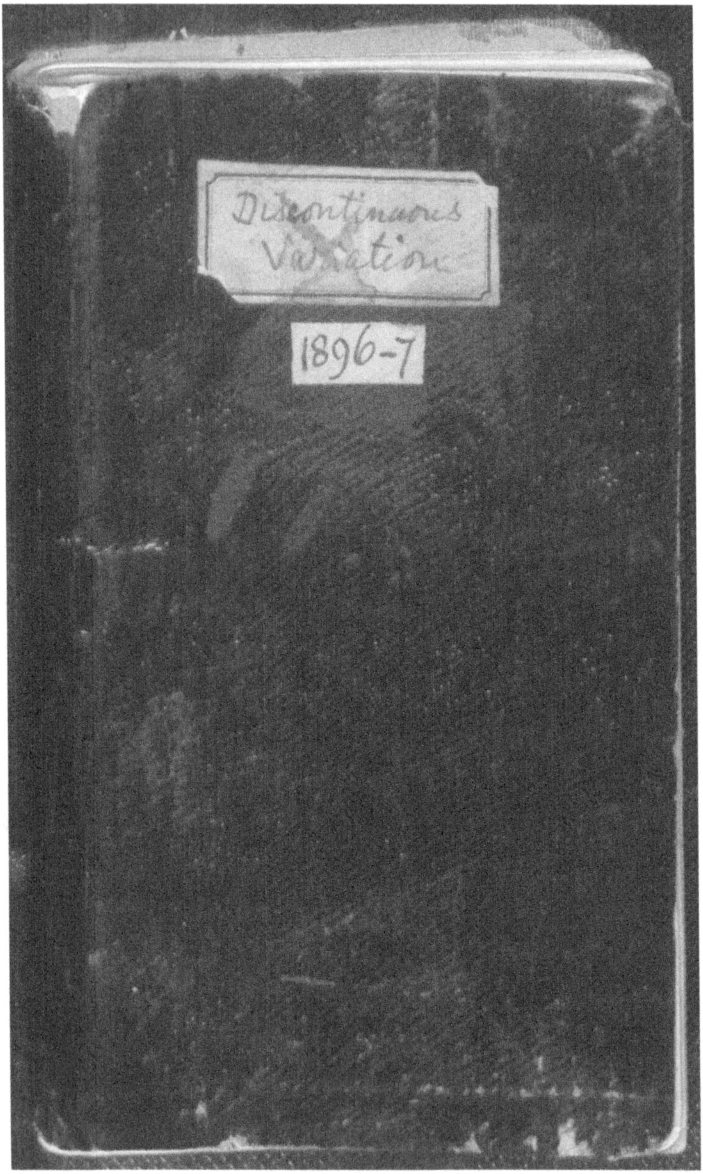

Figure 1.1: The 'Discontinuous Variation' Notebook which contains the Mars story.

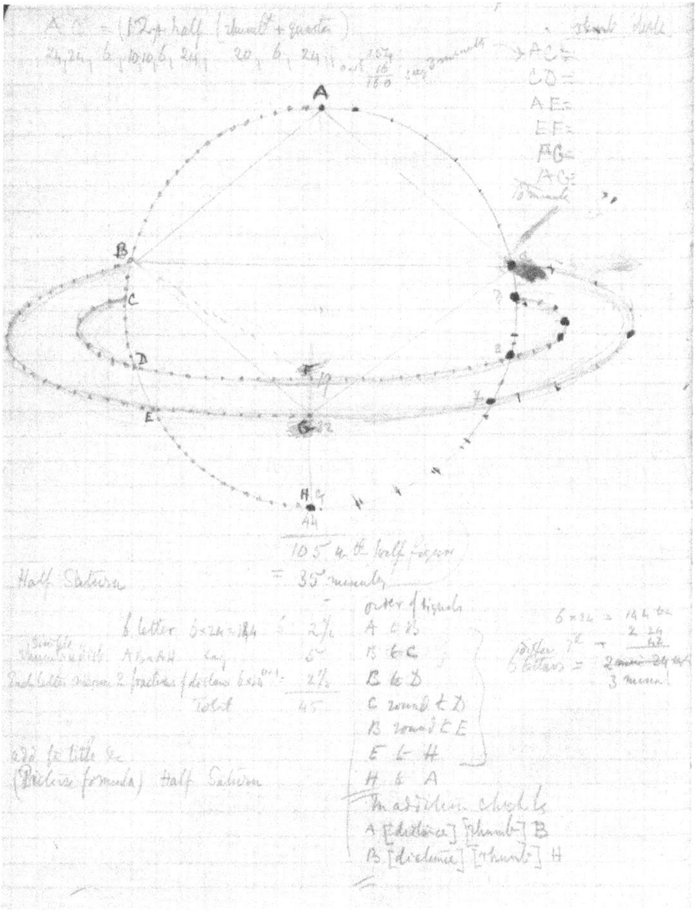

Figure 1.2: Encoding a picture of Saturn for transmission to Mars.

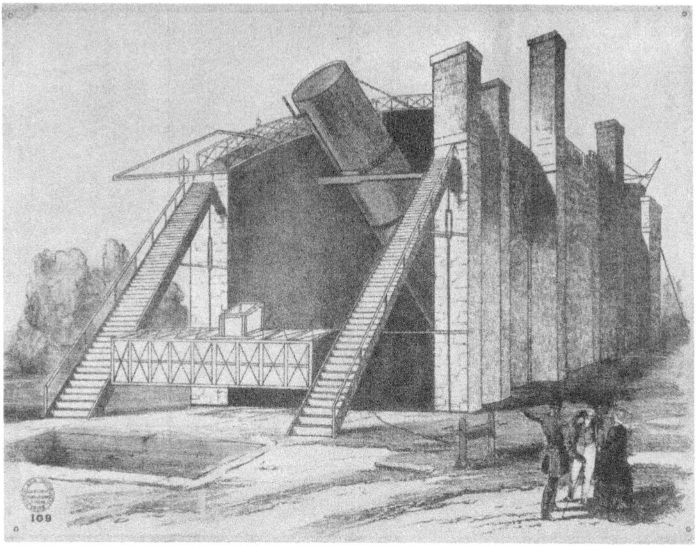

Figure 1.3: *Lord Rosse's Leviathan of Parsonstown.*

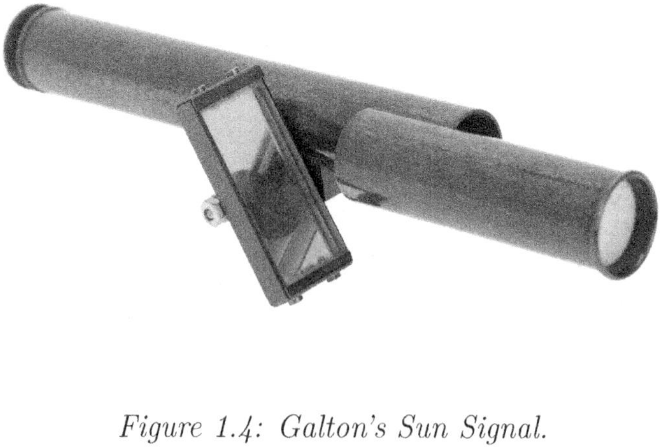

Figure 1.4: *Galton's Sun Signal.*

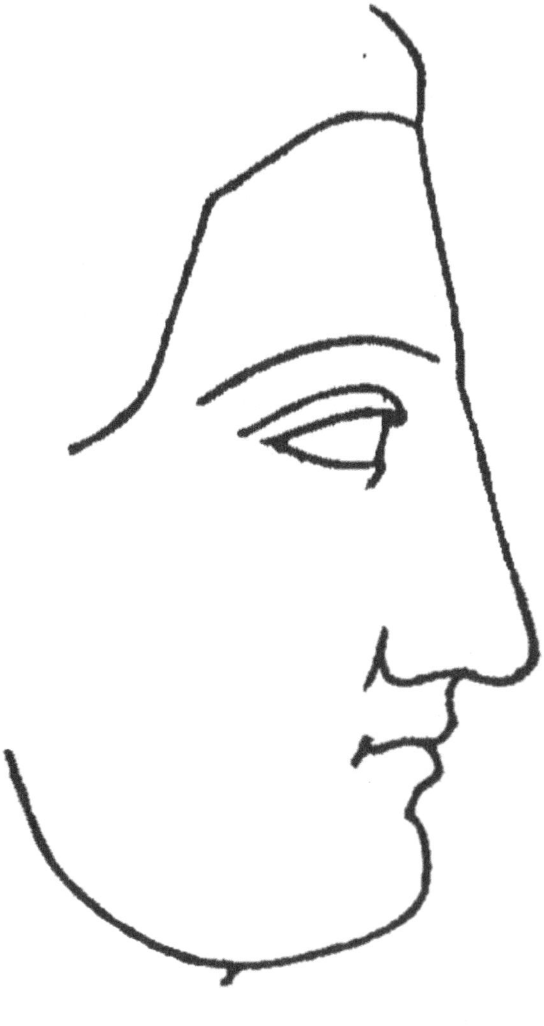

Figure 1.5: Profile of a Greek Girl from a Medallion, for Encoding.

11	**21**	**31**	**41**	**51**	**61**	**71**
12	**22**	**32**	**42**	**52**	**62**	**72**
13	**23**	**33**	**43**	**53**	**63**	**73**
14	**24**	**34**	**44**	**54**	**64**	**74**
15	**25**	**35**	**45**	**55**	**65**	**75**
16	**26**	**36**	**46**	**56**	**66**	**76**
17	**27**	**37**	**47**	**57**	**67**	**77**

Figure 1.6: Grid-based moves. Each successive dot is recentered at 44 for the next move.

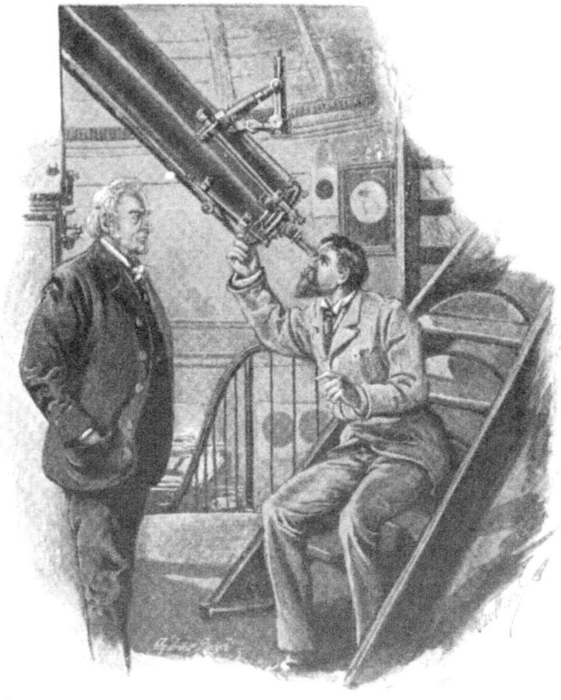

Figure 1.7: Peering at Mars, as imagined by Cassell's Family Magazine *in 1895.*

Chapter 2

Rough Outline

Opportunity approaches sh^{d} be seized (letter by an Amateur) Optimist

Letter by Optimist

Newspaper commentary we are ants, Earth Folk may be quite different, even developed vertebrates without antennae / no intelligible signals possible—just an answering flash, no more useless attempt and very costly as communicated by official astronomer who grumbles

Amateur astronomer. letter. twinklings from bright crescent of Earth like to but more intense than the sun on [blue] they have a [purposive] appearance - request for telesc. 3 times more effective Newsp. after a year or so happy announce that by [bounty] of rich canal proprietor telescope is got mounted & is [nearly] ready for use

Another astron.: there is no doubt now of the telegraphic characters – but no clue yet to their meaning. Each message lasts for about an hour. Signals are made only from one point in the earth & are so timed that none are sent when sun is less than 20°above horizon at that point. Apparatus to record is in hand

Amateur Astron: Frequent failures owing to various accidents including earth clouds &c. but it appears that [the] whole communication consists of different messages one of which is sent every 4 days the others have each one day to themselves. By accumulating the records of 2 or 3 their several deficiencies will soon be made good

Amateur Astron.: Hurrah—the first 2 sets are quite made out & the first gives a clue to all the rest. The results will be communicated today, to the A Soc. The rest is under earnest consideration but puzzles at present.

Newspapers of next day, popular account of numerals & signs & decimal point

Official Astron.: grumbles at decimal system & speculates on its cause

Amateur astron.: announcement of drawing. much remains to be deciphered errors in long series

Newspaper popular account

Amateur astron. announcement of pictures of earth fish, horse, birds, lizards and butterflies

Philosophers letters on female neuters

Male writes a letter

Speculations as to how to reply & carry on the communications

Chapter 3

Introduction

In the following pages will be found a free translation of a series of letters which will appear about the middle of the approaching century in the *Bellona Gazette*, which is the leading newspaper of the planet Mars. The translation is as faithful as practicable, considering the very great differences in conditions of light on Mars and here. The numerical system of the Mars folk, their measures. dates & so forth, are translated into our own. Alas many expressions, which would otherwise be misinterpreted or altogether unintelligible without voluminous explanations, have been terrestialised, so to speak.

This book will of course be of interest to students of the occult sciences and it will also be of great service to them. They have hitherto been unable to satisfy the legitimate demand for proofs of their high professions. That deficiency is here supplied with fullest measure. How indeed, may they triumphantly say, would it be possible to anticipate, by half a century, occurrences on a scene some hundreds of millions of miles away from the earth, without methods which according to the incorrect phraseology of the present day are termed supernatural?

3.1 Preliminary

- 6 legs like centaurs 15 hands high, faces like diver's costume—no hearing — antennae

- Gesture communication like deaf mutes — Oxford chapel[1] — middle limbs

- Neuter females — passion for routine work like women knitting & sewing, love of eggs & larvae — aversion to males, but [cowed] by them also [conscious] of their supremacy all round. Great fear of & respect for fertile females

- Males vivacious warlike, only jealous during brief season of love—chivalrous all poetry, eloquence with gesture, art resided with them. Loyal to fertile females. Indifferent to [undermen] of the neuters

[1] Oxford Street chapel for deaf mutes, see below.

■ Fertile females about 1 to 10 males — House wifery — lay numerous eggs at one season of the year. No care for them — the neuter females do that — They select their males & mate

■ Egg for a short time — then [labor] for 6 months — are watched & tended much as growing crops not loved. A provisional selection of about 1 in 10 is made. The rest killed [survivors] allowed to pupate & the neuters have same passion for the pupae that ants have for theirs. Emergence full grown but soft great anxiety & interest— going to school & college

■ The social system [is] full of interest but will not be touched on here—Many communities, usually at war

■ Mars [Moon] Bellona war battle warrior arms sword spears lance dagger club mace arrow bow sling archer bayonet mail broadsword spur trumpet dram murder homicide fury, [...], hate despair groans, agony, shriek yell blood slaughter wound gash victory conqueror

3.2 Ethnography

The Mars folk resemble ants in many particulars, though far larger and more highly developed. Their fore pair of limbs are equal to any hands in their power of grasp and delicacy of touch, though of course they differ greatly from them in shape.

The Mars folk, as quadrupeds, walk on the middle & hind pairs of limbs with their heads erect & arms fore, bearing a resemblance to small, slightly made & very agile centaurs the same height as the back of a chair. Each of the middle pair of limbs is furnished like those of ants, with a powerful pair of claws. These are of much use to artisans, who rest themselves on the tripod formed by the end of the body & the two hinder limbs, then grasping any object between the claws of the middle pair, as between two vices, their hands are free to operate upon it. Their skeletons are wholly external like a panoply of heavy armour, but its weight is unimportant since the force of gravity on M is only a third of that on the E. Their sense of hearing is almost deficient but their eye power is acute and ample. Their lateral eyes as in ants, are of the mosaic type consisting of a vast number of facets each of which admits a beam of light so narrow that objects are in focus at all ranges, with the result that almost the whole panoramic area is simultaneously in view and no change can occur in the surrounding objects without attracting attention. The folk are therefore even more alive to what is going on around them than our deaf-mutes. They have 3 frontal eyes like ants, of the same order as our own, one of which is highly myopic & serves as strong lens. They are highly developed. In short the optics of the M folk are much more efficient than our own, both in respect to the acuteness of vision, and in the width of their field of view. They see minute & distant objects with the keenness of eagles & squirrels and their unaided eyesight is quite as good as ours when we are aided by an opera glass.

Their senses of taste & especially that of smell are highly discriminative and so is that of the touch in the hand & certain parts of the body, principally through the medium of bristles and hairs which pass through holes in the external armour to the sensitive flesh behind it. But above all the rest in sensitivity of touch are the antennae which [during] conversation between social equals and friends are in constant movement and touch. They convey not only as much as ordinary men & women can convey by grasp, squeezes and gentle pressures of the hand, but quite as much as any 'thought' reader or rather any gesture interpreter can make out from them. Their peculiar power leads to curious customs, one is that in diplomatic conferences where whatever is 'said' (i.e. conveyed by signs) at the council table must be spoken to all, the members are to wear official costume consisting of a sort of helmet with hollow horns to contain & conceal the antennae. Their public utterances are also gesture language like that of deaf mutes, which may be seen in operation any Sunday in the pulpit in the Deaf Mute chapel in Oxford street. It is easily understood that their [physiognomies] & faces are not in the least what we should call beautiful; they roughly resemble that of a diver in full costume.

The people are divided, as ants are, into 3 principal groups: the fertile females, males, and neuter females, but their proportionate numbers differ considerably. In the same community there are usually many fertile females, which is rarely the case in ants (——[2] being one of the few exceptions) and attached to each of these there [are] half a dozen or a dozen males. The season of love is of brief duration and at other times of the year social life proceeds calmly even among the males, though they are always apt to fight on slight questions of honour.

Life is begun in the form of an egg the size of that of a hen or a crocodile which is laid about a fortnight after the close of the mating season. Each fertile female lays a large number of them in rather quick suc-

[2] Omitted by Galton.

cession with small strain to her health & strength. Afterwards she cares no more about the eggs, but returns to her usual & queenly & housewifely life, while they are looked after by the neuter females. In another week's time, the larvae are hatched which are about 6 inches long at first. They are tended with great care by the neuters who assiduously note & record [the] physical & instinctive peculiarities of each larva, with the view of determining which should ultimately preserved and which destroyed. Perhaps 20 times as many larvae [leave] the egg as are allowed to pupate. The attachment of the neuter nurses to the larvae is of a curious business-like kind, there is no love in it, for these neuter females seem incapable of true affection. Anyhow they nurse, watch & observe the larvae sedulously, and from time to time a formal consultation takes place between the queen & males, after which the neuters kill quite coolly those of their growing charges who it has been judged undesirable to preserve.

Some few unpromising larvae are always kept for scientific investigation, to see how they will turn out in after life, it being of obvious importance to the community that the selected larvae should really be the fittest and it is only by careful test experiments that the value of the rules under which the selection takes place can be confirmed & the rules themselves gradually improved. The larvae lead a purely animal existence feeding & fattening enormously; their numbers are from time to time reduced as above described until at the time of pupation 12 months after they began to live; there remain but only nine that are intended to live, each being a huge grub some 4 feet long & six or 7 inches thick.

When the larvae show signs of approaching pupation they are placed into separate cells where they weave a cocoon about themselves. There they lie, with little help, outwardly impassive but inwardly undergoing rapid & continuous changes, until the time comes that they burst their cases, aided by anxious neuters, and emerge feeble & limp but as perfectly good M folk, so far as physical form is concerned. There follows a long period of hardening and what may be called school & college life, after which certain probationary tests with accompanying ceremonies are gone through, and the probationaries receive the full rights of citizenship.

It w^{d} take far more space than can now be spared to describe the social life, so different from our own, of these communities, whose stability rests largely on the division of their constituents. The fertile females queen it over the males. They are superior to any one of them in size & strength and such is the constitution of the sexes that while their figures & demeanour excite some fear in the weaker males, they also evoke their chivalrous loyalty and attachment The fertile females rarely associate; they do not necessarily dislike one another but they are too jealous & self-contained for mutual friendship. Each keeps her own court and they intercommunicate by usually neuter agents.

The neuter females possess no [quality] that we should call loveable; they are devoid of heart & generosity & they have but little originality—but they continually occupy themselves with work of some sort however [measly] & cannot keep still for a moment. Whatever passion they possess is socialistic—they certainly care little for themselves and much for the community, and though very obstinate in small things are practically directed by the males, with the concurrence of the queens, towards whom their attitude of mind is [...] It is one neither of personal love nor of personal loyalty, but rather one of respect for the temporary representatives of a [caste] which prevents the community from becoming extinct, by replenishing it through their eggs.

The males are warriors. They have all of the truly male virtues and all the manly defects of our race; they are the salt of the community both morally & intellectually. They look on the neuters as 'hands' in a factory, not particularly disliking or contemning them, but as members of a different social stratum, who have to be dealt with in matters of business, but not as friends. In the course of history, rebellions of the neuters have occurred, nearly all of which the rapid and concentrated action of the warlike males have achieved [...] often bloody victories over, with the result that queens & males have taken good care that the number of neuter pupae should be kept as low as national convenience would permit, for future generations.

That part of their civilization which will chiefly concern us is the mechanical & mathematical side which is fully as much developed among their professionals as among our own. As the laws & materials of nature are much the same throughout the solar system, their inventions are to a considerable extent parallel to our own though different in details, but their ethics are altogether of another kind. Their consciences are not like ours, nor are their chief pleasures & ambitions like those by which we are moved. They are far more alien to us than the Chinese & that is saying not a little. Into these interesting psychological topics we must not enter now, for they have no direct bearing on the work before us.

Chapter 4

Extracts from the *Bellona Gazette*

4.1 Letter from Optimist

Sir. Before many months are over, Mars & the Earth will make their nearest approach & Mars will appear to the earth folk as a brilliant planet, shining during the whole of many of their successive nights. I urge again, as others have urged on previous similar occasions, to seize this admirable opportunity of endeavouring to transmit some visible signals to our nearest neighbour. We might be able for example to flash a huge sun signal to them, to which they might subsequently respond when the earth had moved so far from the direct line between Mars & the sun as to re-appear as a luminous crescent. In short the Earth might signal to us pretty freely during the beginning of her first quarter & towards the close of her third quarter. She would then be at from about —— to —— millions of miles from us; far indeed but not too far for the purpose. The cost and magnitude of the signalling would of course be very great, but not insurmountable. If we consider on the one hand the acres of glass used for corridors of hot houses it seems not at all unreasonable to hope that some practical scheme might be worked out by which thousands of separated mirrors, each of them under the charge of two men, might be simultaneously worked [...] under the orders of 2 fuglemen,[1] one of whom should indicate the direction & the other the duration of the flashes. Men [who] a flourishing community had no particular use for [...] and who desired to make themselves famous, might be disposed to carry through the undertaking.

Optimist.

4.2 Letter from *Respice Finem* [Consider the consequences].

I will not enter in to the [imperfect] consideration whether the proposed signals could really as explained be made, but wish to point out that at the best [their] value would be very small. The result could only be

[1] Drill models for showing how things are to be done.

that we had made a signal & that the Earth had reciprocated it, proving that the earth was inhabited by observant & intelligent beings. Very probably it is [so] but the fact would be placed beyond doubt by this experiment. This however is the sum total of what we could possibly learn. We & the Earth folk have no common language or means of forming one & consequently no means can exist for rational communication. We could never learn what we most want to know such as the forms & features of the inhabitants of the earth, their industries and inventions, their social life, the exact amount of their intelligence & so forth. If it were possible to learn all or a part of this, a costly experiment might be reasonably undertaken by zealous men, but all the knowledge that we could achieve is so ludicrously inferior to this that the proposed experiment could not be other than a piece of wasteful folly.

Respice Finem.

4.3 Letter from "Common Sense"

Sir. A prospect such as that in the letter of Optimist is almost too absurd for a philosopher to notice, but as enthusiasm is catching, and as you have probably many readers who are both ignorant & of an enthusiastic temperament I beg to submit a few common sense considerations before they are led away by [foolish] [notions].

First, supposing the [unnecessarily] costly apparatus to have been made and the double thousands of men to have been obtained, paid for & instructed to work it, and again that the Earth folk would follow suit, what at the best could it lead to? We should learn that Earth was inhabited by observant mechanical creatures, having some understanding; but beyond that nothing. Mars would have, so to speak, waved something; Earth after the lapse of some weeks or months would have waved in reply.

Our knowledge of the Earth folk would go no further. It would clearly be impossible to communicate further in an intelligible way, even if signalling [to & fro] were prompt, for we can invent no common language. Even under the most favourable suppositions the costly undertaking would lead to almost nothing. On the other hand the probability that the earth is inhabited by creatures who could & would reply is infinitesimally small. Its animals and plants must differ wildly from our own and however various & numerous they may be, it is scarcely likely that any one of them should have arrived at the mental stature of Mars folk, who are the Lords of all living things in their planet. Yet the students of evolution prove that we Mars folk are mere varieties of the common ant and collateral descendants from a common stock. Ants have six limbs like ourselves, though their middle pair are shorter, the hard skeleton that supports their frame like ours is external; their populations are divided into fertile females, males, and working neuters and so are ours, though by no means in the same proportions. The only really novel point in our structure is the arrangement for expelling air through a reed like structure in various ways, that is capable or producing a variety of sounds combined with a complex auditory apparatus by which those sounds can be heard & distinguished.

We and the ants are alike provided with at least five principal senses, that is we see, feel, taste and smell; and the antenna-tact. Therefore although we are vastly larger than they are, measuring fully 4 feet in height when we assume the ordinary posture of the insect, and although our mouths are far less prognathous than theirs & shapely & expressive and although our fore pair of limbs are furnished with delicate apparatus for touch and handling & our middle pair are reduced to powerful [holders] these details do not affect the essential similarity. When one of our artisans sits on the ground, stayed by his [diverging] legs, and [grasps] an object between the claws of his middle limbs, as in a vice, while he operates upon it with his hands, he looks at a distance very like an ant. How can we expect that the evolution of the Earth folk should have followed the same particular line as that of our ancestors? Nay, why should this structure have originated in an insect form? It is conceivable for instance that the vertebrate class of animals may have capacities for development and that the ruling earth folk may be related to the agile & mischievous monkey or to the slow obstinate ass. Any how it is most improbable that the ruling Earth Folk, if such there be, should have any features, thoughts & feelings in common with ourselves that would make rational intercommunication possible. If a community of Mars Folk runs mad & chooses to spend their [overplus] fortune in carrying out the proposal of "Optimist" then the name of that community will undoubtedly be handed down in future generations as the perpetrators of a most egregious piece of folly.

Yours &c. Common Sense.

4.4 Letter from Bellona Observatory

Certain phenomena on the surface of the earth have been under careful observation by my assistants for some time past, signs which require very careful investigation with a more powerful telescope than this observatory has at its disposal. It is well known that a small luminous spot is often visible on the globe of this planet, caused by the reflection of the sun from the face of one of the seas when the water is calm, and the sky clear. The phenomenon about which I am about to speak is also a luminous speck but distinctly smaller & more intense. It proceeds from the same definite part of the Earth's surface which is certainly not sea, on apparently a high plateau situated in the neighbourhood of what appears to be tracts of snow in the subtropical region. It is also noticeable that the point in question is one that for a long time past has been described by astronomers as rarely hidden by clouds, and therefore may have been selected as appropriate for making these signals. This luminous speck flickers at various rates and apparently in a purposive way, just as though an attempt were being made by the Earth folk to attract our notice by flashing sun signals. It appears to me, from experiments I have made on the visibility of sun signals, that a telescope of double, preferably of treble, the efficiency of the largest under my control would be adequate to carry out the desired investigation. I am doing my best to obtain funds for the construction of such a telescope. It would not be extremely costly as some delicacy of definition might be sacrificed in order to procure the needful amount of illumination and magnifying power.

Bellona Observatory

4.5 Paragraph from the *Bellona Gazette*

We are able with much pleasure to announce that all the parts of the huge telescope are completed. They are now being put together with much rapidity, and unless some unexpected difficulty should occur the telescope will be in working order in a few days and a commencement made in the study of the very curious scintillations lately observed at one spot in the surface of the earth. Since their occurrence was first publicly announced in these columns by the Director of the Bellona observatory they have been observed by every other astronomer who possesses a good telescope so that the scientific world has become greatly excited by this very strange phenomenon, which there is every reason to believe that the new telescope will succeed in investigating it much more thoroughly than has hitherto been possible.

4.6 Editor of the *Bellona Gazette.*

We are pleased to announce that all the parts of the huge telescope that has been under construction for the Bellona Observatory during several months are made. They are [rapidly being tried] and promise to give every satisfaction. The telescope will very shortly be in readiness for investigating the curious scintillations on the surface of the Earth which still continue. They have been observed by numerous astronomers since their existence was first pointed out in these columns by the Astronomer Royal. The results to be desired from the new telescope are awaited with the keenest anxiety by all scientific men, and will from time to time be announced in these columns.

4.7 Report (a) from the Astronomer of the Bellona Observatory

In anticipation of the appearance in print of a preliminary report just made by me to the Board of Directors, I send by their permission the following extracts to you for publication.

Astronomer, Bell: Obs:

The new telescope fulfils my best expectations and

enables the flashes from the surface of the earth to be clearly seen. They are undoubtedly signals directed to ourselves but I have as yet no clue to decipher them. They consist of what may be called messages that last for an hour or so. Each message consists apparently of words, separated from one another by intervals of 4 seconds. Each word is composed of 1, 2, 3, 4 or 5 signals as the case may be, and these signals are severally short, medium, or long flashes differently arranged to form different words. The intervals between these signals in the same word are of $1\frac{1}{2}$ second duration. Those between the words are 4 seconds, the short signal is of the same length, the medium occupies 3 seconds and the long 5 seconds. The difficulty of accurately recording the signals will soon be got over by a simple instrument now under construction. It is a cylinder covered with paper that revolves slowly by clockwork on an axis. A pencil at the end of a hinge is pressed during the duration of each flash. Thus a spiral record is left on the cylinder of all that has been seen, which can be studied at pleasure. The manuscript records already made are, I regret to say, very imperfect. This was owing to a multitude of small inadvertent accidents which need not occur again. Thus far it appears that one of the messages has already recurred twice [at intervals of] 4 days, but there has as yet been no observed recurrence of each of the others. I gather from this that the series of messages is small and and that the rest of the messages are repeated to make more sure of their being all observed & that the one which is the most often repeated contains the clue to deciphering others. Deficiencies in any record of a message will probably be made good when it is seen a second & third time, so the records of the frequently repeated message will be quite ready for study, and the remainder will be equally well revised & corrected before long.

Chapter 5

Deciphered Messages

5.1 Editorial Paragraph in 2nd Edition Special

A meeting of the Bellona physical society has been hastily convened this evening, the prospect of which is exciting the most extraordinary interest. It is alleged that [the] message that has been the most frequently repeated has been completely deciphered & that [a] full description of the sparkles & of their meaning will be given tonight by the Communal Astronomer.

5.2 Decipherment of a message from the earth

[Article newspaper (Large type heading).]

The wildest anticipations of the scientific men who attended the meeting of last night were fully realised. The room was crowded to excess and the antennae of all present were in the most restless agitation. The illustrations by the lanthorn showed [that] every one of the phrases in the first message, which were so distinctly & yet [simply] arranged that their interpretation was obvious, is necessary. The result is that the symbols are positively determined which the earth folk use to express any desired numeral, for that of equal and for the several operations of addition, subtraction, multiplication & division. The method employed by the Earth Folk is simple & best explained as below, in which the word that apparently corresponds to any given signal is printed in italics & brackets. There is no need to puzzle the reader by printing all the symbols in their actual form, a sample of them will suffice. Thus '....' is found to stand for 4. Each message has a heading, which for the moment we will [ignore] This heading is followed in the first message by (this takes 10 minutes not more)

.	(equal) (one)	.	=	..
..	(equal) (two)	..	=	.-
...	(equal) (three)	...	=	.—
		....	=	-.
		.....	=	- -
	&c. up to 10			

The desire to satisfy the eagerness of the public to hear of any results obtained by the new telescope justifies the recent preliminary account, after only [...] day's experience. It will be shown [...] what has been thus far ascertained with certainty concerning the scintillations and what little has been inferred as to their motive & meaning.

In the first place they are unquestionably made by reasonable beings not by only chance action. There are 3 and only 3 variations of flashes that is of what may be inferred letters which are of short, medium, and long duration, lasting respectively $1\frac{1}{2}$, 3 & 5 seconds. These are formed into what may be called words consisting of 1, 2, 3, 4, 5 letters each, the pause between each letter in the same word being $\frac{1}{2}$ second & that between two succeeding words being 3 seconds. Thus sentences are formed, separated by pauses of 5 seconds or more. Lastly a group of sentences make the nightly message, which lasts about an hour. The messages differ on successive nights and appear to form a cycle. Some [of] the messages certainly recur, but it is premature to say whether all do. The records of what was observed at first are not so trustworthy as is desirable; different plans have been tried with varying success, now however a recording apparatus has been constructed which works quite satisfactorily & gives a duplicate copy. A cylinder covered with two sheets of paper, with carbonised paper interposed revolves by clock work on a long screw for its axis so that a pencil pressed steady on it would leave a continuous spiral trace. The pencil is however mounted on a spring, so that when the finger ceased to press no mark is left. The [observer] has merely to apply his finger whenever & for so long as he sees a flash & the result is a perfect record in the language of dot dash & line.

The question arises what does it all mean? It is a curious fact that the most labored messages consist almost wholly of words of 3 letters. There are some 150 or 200 of these in a single message forming one continuous sentence which is nearly the whole of the message. Now there are only 27 possible varieties of the words formed of the various possible changes of the three letters dot, dash & line (let us say a, b & c). Why are these 27 signals so largely used to the exclusion of all others? No reply has yet suggested itself. A faint clue has presented itself in another direction. Each message has what may be called a heading of two words. The second of these is always the same; it is a word of four letters. The first word differs in successive messages and always consists of two letters. These disyllabic words

so far as they have been recorded formed part of an orderly series of permutations, as follows in which the missing observations are supplied by hypothesis and are for distinction sake printed in italic letters

aa, ab, ac, ba, bc, bd, ca, cd, cd, aa, ab, ac, ba

It certainly looks as though they stood for numerals and that the headings should be read as 'first message', 'second message', 'third message' &c. If this be true, the imperfection of the record [is] the cause why a decipherment of the rest seems impossible. In due course the first message will be repeated in a few days after which we shall be in a better position to theorize than we are at present.

5.3 Complete decipherment of Message 1 from the Earth

It was mentioned in my last letter that imperfections in the record of what was supposed & is now known to be message no. 1 were the reason why the meaning of the signalling generally was at that time undecipherable. The message has again been sent & accurately observed & recorded & its signification is now thoroughly established, and we are already in possession of the meaning of no less than —— different words used by the Earth people.

The bases of their first message are the plain facts of simple arithmetic, by means of which the names of the numerals are defined and the usual symbols of equal, plus, minus, multiplication, addition & the like are fixed. Any misgiving that may remain about the true interpretation of any of these will almost certainly be cleared away as the decipherment of the remaining messages proceeds.

Suppose a person first to make one flash, then after a pause to make two flashes, then three, & so on; there could be little doubt that he was following the numerals in their natural order of 1 2 3 &c. This with a little variation from the beginning of the first message [is] as follows

.	-	. .
. .	-	. -
. . .	-	. -
. . . .	-	- .
. . . . .	-	- -
. . . . . .	-	- —
. . . .	-	— .
. . . .	-	— -
. . . .	-	— —

The '-' in the middle of each entry stands we may presume for 'equal to' and the last word for the numeral. This presumption is turned into certainty by the next group of sentences. Here & for the future in order to avoid puzzling the reader with dots, dashes & lines, the presumed word or phrase will be printed in italics within brackets. When the word or phrase has been established it will be printed in ordinary type within brackets.

The second group of sentences is of this form, a new word of 4 letters which is interpreted as plus makes its appearance in them.

(1) (plus) (1) (equal to) (2); (2) (plus) (3) (equal to) (5); & so on for—— sentences. There can now be no doubt as to the correctness of the interpretation; certainly none remains after the third group of (2) (minus) (1) (equal to) (1); (4) (minus) (1) (equal to)

(3) &c.

So the numerals 1 to 9 and the signs 'equal', 'plus' & 'minus' have been communicated & established through some 30 minutes of signalling. The same process explains the signs for multiplication, twice 2 = 4, twice 3 = 6, twice 4 = 8, thrice 3 = 9. Similarly as to the sign for division.

Thus far the numerals 1 to 9 have alone been used. The next group of sentences gives 0 and extends the system of numeration indefinitely, by the method of notation familiar to us, with the exception that it is decimal and not octessimal. The octessimal is common to all communities of Mars folk; doubtless because we have 8 members all told, our 6 limbs & 2 antennae. It is a passable method, though inferior to the duodecimal; in view of the great trouble of making a change to [it] we have continued its use, but the decimal system of notation is ludicrously bad, the number 10 being divisible only by 2 & by 5, whereas 12 is divisible by 2, 3, 4 & 6. It is not however to be supposed that the earth folk use such an absurd system for their own purposes, but that they have translated their own notation into it on account of the convenience of the nine variations in words of 2 letters. It seems certain that their own system cannot be [octessimal] like ours, otherwise the nine variations would have exactly suited a 0 and 8 numerals. It has been jokingly suggested that the earth folk may be developed vertebrates [having] five digits to each hand, like the monkey, & that the decimal system may be founded on that fact, but it would be a waste of time to dwell on such fancies.

The sentences in question are these $9 + 1 = 10$, $9 + 2 = 11$, $9 + 3 = 12$, (&c., and again $10 \times 2 = 20$, $10 \times 3 = 30$, $10 \times 10 = 100$, $100 \times 10 = 1000$, (&c. The word interpreted as '&c. is a succession of 5 dots; which interpretation will be confirmed directly. The concluding group of sentences given the significance (decimal point) suggests that of (approximately) and confirms the &c. It is by such sentences as 7 (divided by $2 = 3.5$; 7 divided by 3 2.33333 (&c. =2.3 (approximately), 5 divided by $4 =$ (1.25) 8 (divided by) $3 = 2.66666$ (&c. $= 2.7$ (approximately)

A final sentence defines briefer symbols for $\frac{1}{2}$ & $\frac{1}{4}$, they are of 3 letters each and become of use later on. This concludes the first message which occupies a little less than 1 hour in its delivery. It is obvious that if we in Mars were in position to flash back replies to the earth, the foundation is laid for any amount of algebraic intercommunication, but let it not be supposed for a moment that the earth can talk to us only about arithmetic & algebra. There is much more coming upon which I hope to make a further communication very shortly

The sentences in the earlier message consist usually of five words only several occupy on the average about $1\frac{1}{4}$ minute, thus between 40 & 50 of them are transmitted in one hour.

It is a curious feature that some of the messages consist mainly of words of only 2 letters & others of words of only 3 letters, though from the nature of the case there can be but 6 varieties of the former & 27 of the latter.[1]

5.4 Decipherment of the second message from the earth

In this message certain names are established apparently for further use in building up a common language. The first group of sentences give the names of the sun & principal planets, namely Venus, Earth, Mars, Jupiter & Saturn, by a method that every astronomer would quickly discover. Their relative mean distance from the sun, their diameters, time of revolution round their several axes are familiar data, as well as much else, but the earth signals are only concerned with these. They are as follows (diameter of) (Sun) & ... & (diameter of) (Venus) (diameter of) (Mars) & ... & (diameter of) (Earth) & ... & (diameter of) (Jupiter) ...; (diameter of) (Saturn)

[1] Stray text: The messages.

Their sequence of numbers is sufficient to establish the words in brackets [as] the names of the planets again appear in similar sentences referring to their mean distances from the sun, all in terms of the earth's diameter as a unit. Our astronomers of course know the length of this in our own measures, so a unit of length is established between us and the earth. The sentences seen thus (Sun) (mean distance from of) (Venus); (Sun) (mean distance from of) (Mars) &c. Similar sentences give a unit of time in terms of one rotation of the earth round its axis thus (sun) (time of rotation round its axis) 25 .. (Venus) (time of rotation round its axis).

This group of sentences occupies 24 minutes

The next group in the second message occupies 25 minutes [and] is comparatively uninteresting in itself, but is a necessary step towards the extraordinary information that we shall have to describe in the next letter & which is not yet wholly deciphered. The delay is not owing to want of clue, but simply to want of time, just as a long despatch in cipher requires time to write out & verify. The data we are now speaking of are the names of a circle and of regular polygons of 3, 4, 5, 6, 7, 8, 9, 10, 12, & 24 sides respectively, including the words circumference, area of (radius of)

The first sentence shows the well-known relation of the circumference of a circle to its diameter, commonly written π thus (π) = 3.1415927

(circle) (circumference of)	=	2π r (area of)	=	π x r x r
(triangle) (circumference of)	=	3s (area of)	=	0.433 &c.
(square) (circumference of)	=	4s	=	1.000
		5s	=	1.720
		6		2.598
		7s		4.828
		9		6.181
		10		7.694
		12		11.196
		24		45.68 about

It is perhaps needless to say that the sides of the figures are in each case taken as units, otherwise of the side be s the above well-known figures have to be multiplied by s^2

5.5 Decipherment of the third message

Strange as it may seem, the earth folk have actually contrived a plan of communicating drawings. They have converted the elements of units in the third message and have sent an excellent drawing of Saturn with 5 rings. It is to these drawings that one half of the long sentences refer which, consisting of words of 3 letters. There are 27 different combinations of the letters but of these the first 24 are alone used, the [last] 3 namely (— — ·) (— — -) (— — —) being omitted.[2]

The 24 are used to specify lines that are respectively parallel and equal to those of a regular polygon of 24 sides, or let us say stitches of equal length such as are used in embroidery, which are parallel to those sides, and inclined each to its predecessor by successive steps of the 24th part of a circle, that is of 15°. Thus (· · ·) may be supposed to represent a stitch directed to the North, the next stitch (· · -) is directed 30 ° to the East side of North, (· · —) is 45° on the East side of North, & so on, until we come to the 23rd side which is (— - —) After which

[2] Ed. The last three words are used as length fractions. Brackets have been added to delimit signal words from punctuation more clearly in the text.

the cycle recommences at the 24th or the 0th side whichever we please to call it & which is as already said (· · ·) The number 24 has unquestionably been selected by the Earth folk on account of its divisibility by many different factors, namely by 2, 3, 4, 6, 8 & 12, whereas 27 is divisible only by 3 and 9 and is not capable of the expressing of a right angle. The division of a circle [into] 24 parts is delicate enough for ordinary purposes but occasionally a decimal may be used to divide the angular interspaces into parts of 1°30'. Again the stitches may when desired be reduced one quarter, one half, or three quarters of their lengths by adding one or other of the 3 omitted symbols. The power of doing this is [...] the contour takes a quick turn, too quick to be expressed by stitches of the same length as those used for the rest of the drawing.

The method by which the process is explained is by signalling (24-gon) (· · ·) (· · -) (· · —) (· - ·) (· - —) & so on to the 23d or 0th side then follows (12-gon) (· · ·) (· · -) (· · —) (· - ·) & so on round to (· · ·), then (8-on) (6-gon) (4-gon) & (3-gon) all in the same way. After this varieties are given of the (3-gon) a few of the (4-gon) fewer of the (6-gon) &c. (thus for under ½ hour) Here follows ½ Saturn [...].[3] 38

[3] Ed. See Figure 1.2, p. 23.

minutes letters & all.[4]

[4] Ed. Transmission time. Annotated by Galton: 'give the complete signal'.

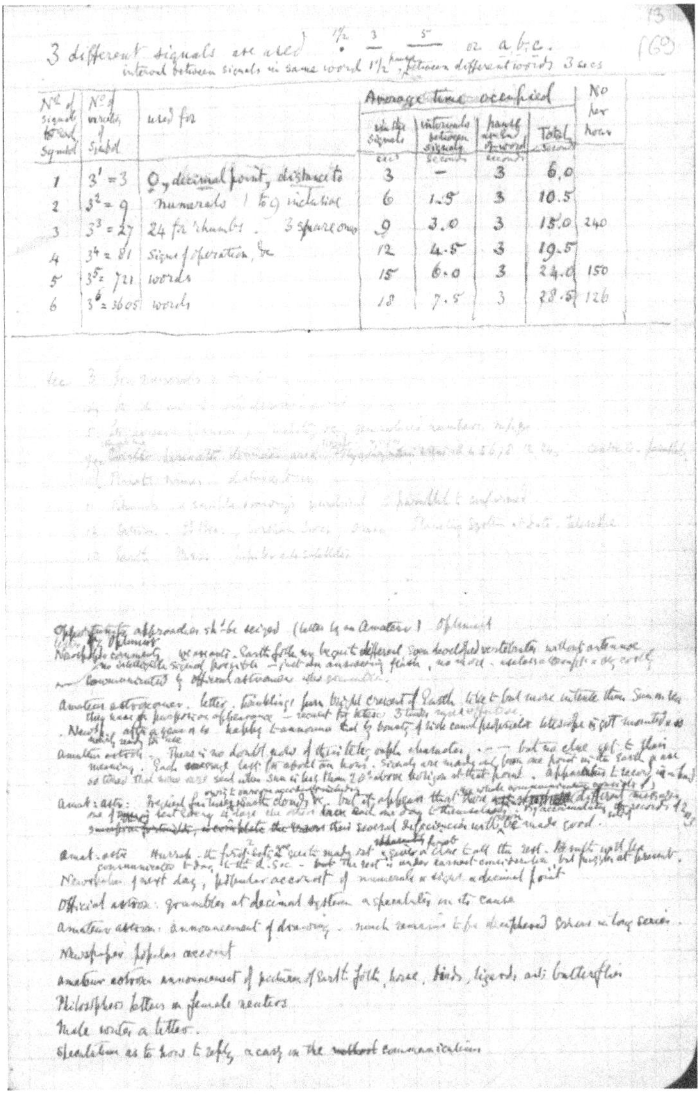

3 different signals are used · — — or a, b, c.

interval between signals in same word 1½, between different words 3 secs

No. of signals to each symbol	No. of varieties of symbol	used for	Average time occupied: in the signals	intervals between signals	pause ... word	Total seconds	No per hour
1	$3^1 = 3$	0, decimal point, distance to	3	—	3	6.0	
2	$3^2 = 9$	numerals 1 to 9 notation	6	1.5	3	10.5	
3	$3^3 = 27$	24 for [illegible]. 3 spare ones	9	3.0	3	15.0	240
4	$3^4 = 81$	Signs of operation, &c	12	4.5	3	19.5	
5	$3^5 = 721$	words	15	6.0	3	24.0	150
6	$3^6 = 3605$	words	18	7.5	3	28.5	126

Official astron: grumbles at decimal system & speculates on its cause

Amateur astron: announcement of drawing. much remains to be deciphered. Others in long series.

Newspaper popular account

Amateur astron: announcement of picture of Earth folk, horse, birds, lizards and butterflies

Philosophers letters on female readers

Male writes a letter.

Speculation as to how to reply, a craze on the communication

Figure 5.1: Page 13 of the Notebook.

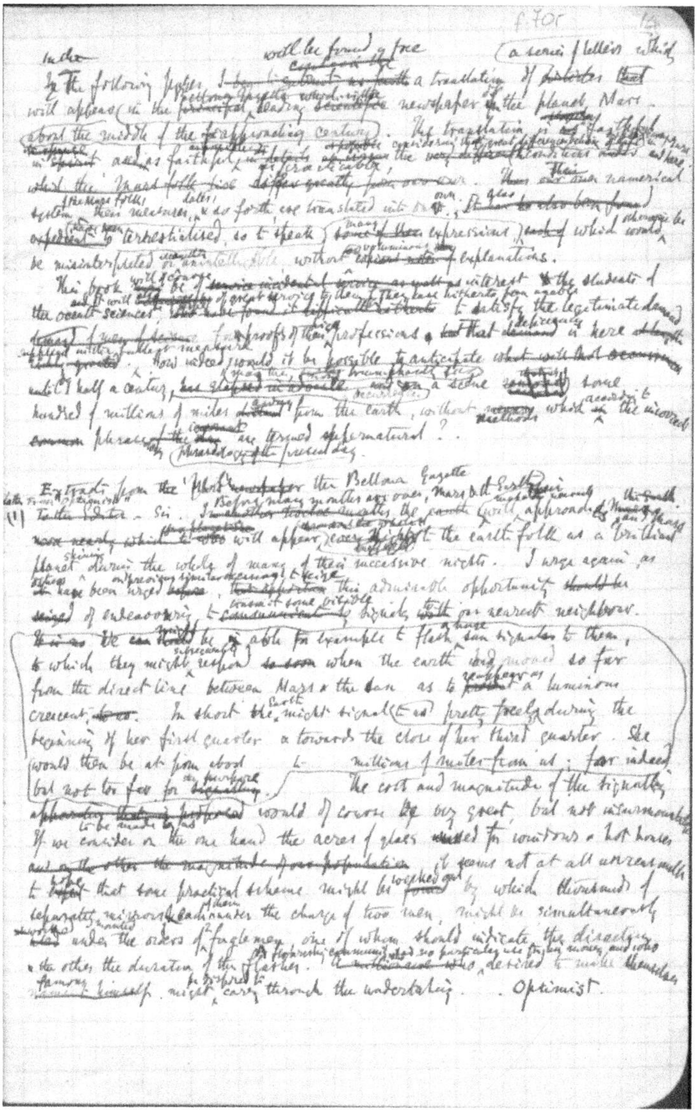

Figure 5.2: Page 14 of the Notebook.

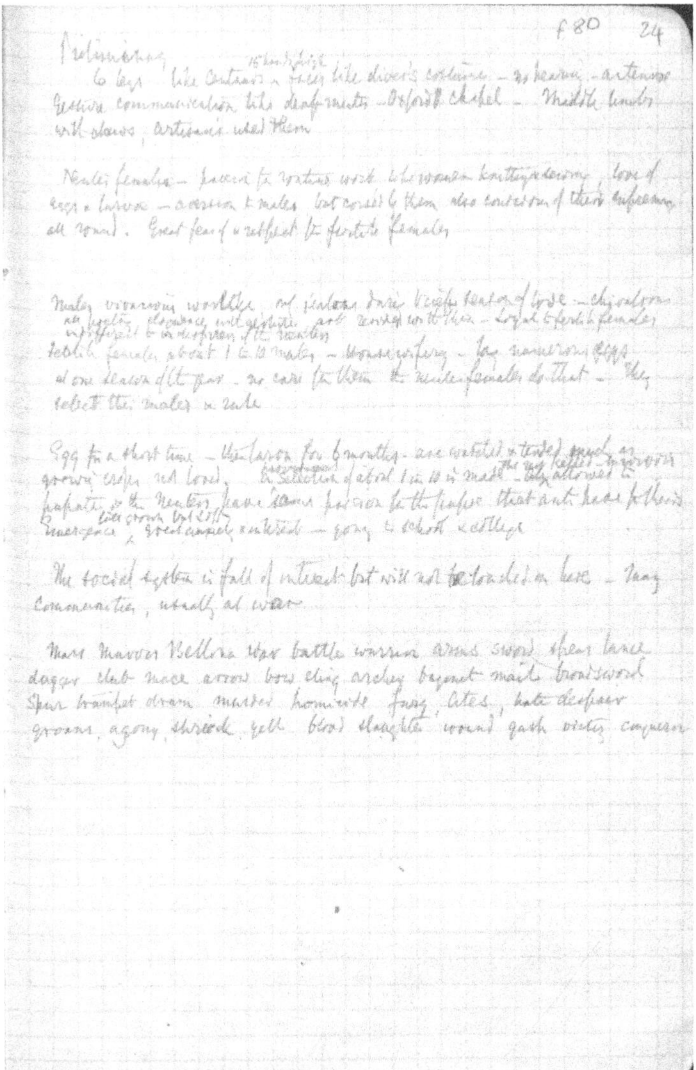

f 80 24

Preliminary

6 legs like Centaurs – faces like diver's costume – no hearing – antennae. Gesture communication like deaf-mutes – Oxford chapel – Middle limbs with claws, artisans used them

Neuter females – [illegible] for [illegible] work like women knitting & sewing – love of eggs & larvae – aversion to males but [illegible] to them also [illegible] of their [illegible] all round. Great fear of & respect for fertile females

Males [illegible] warlike [illegible] jealous [illegible] season of love – chivalrous – no [illegible] [illegible] – Loyal to fertile females – indifferent to [illegible] of the neuters

fertile females about 1 to 10 males – housewifery – lay numerous eggs at one season of the year – no care for them the neuter females do that – they select the males & [illegible]

Egg for a short time – the larva for 6 months – are watched & tended much as growing crops [illegible] [illegible]. [illegible] Selection of about 1 in 10 is made – the rest killed – [illegible] allowed to [illegible] & the neuters have same [illegible] for the [illegible] that ants have for their emergence, [illegible] great anxiety & [illegible] – going to school & college

The social system is full of interest but will not be touched on here – Many communities, usually at war

Mars Mavors Bellona War battle warrior arms sword spear lance dagger club mace arrow bow sling archery bayonet mail broadsword Spur trumpet drum murder homicide fury, [illegible], hate despair groans, agony, shriek, yell blood slaughter wound gash victory conquer

Figure 5.3: Page 24 of the Notebook.

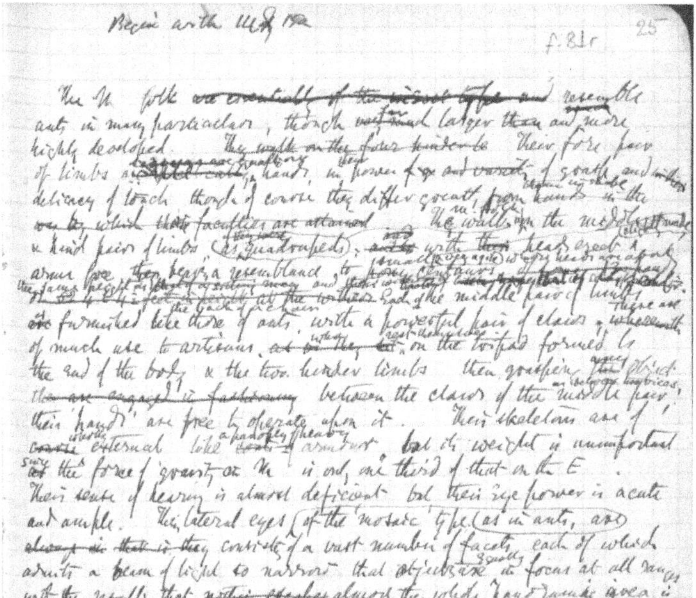

Figure 5.4: Page 25 of the Notebook.

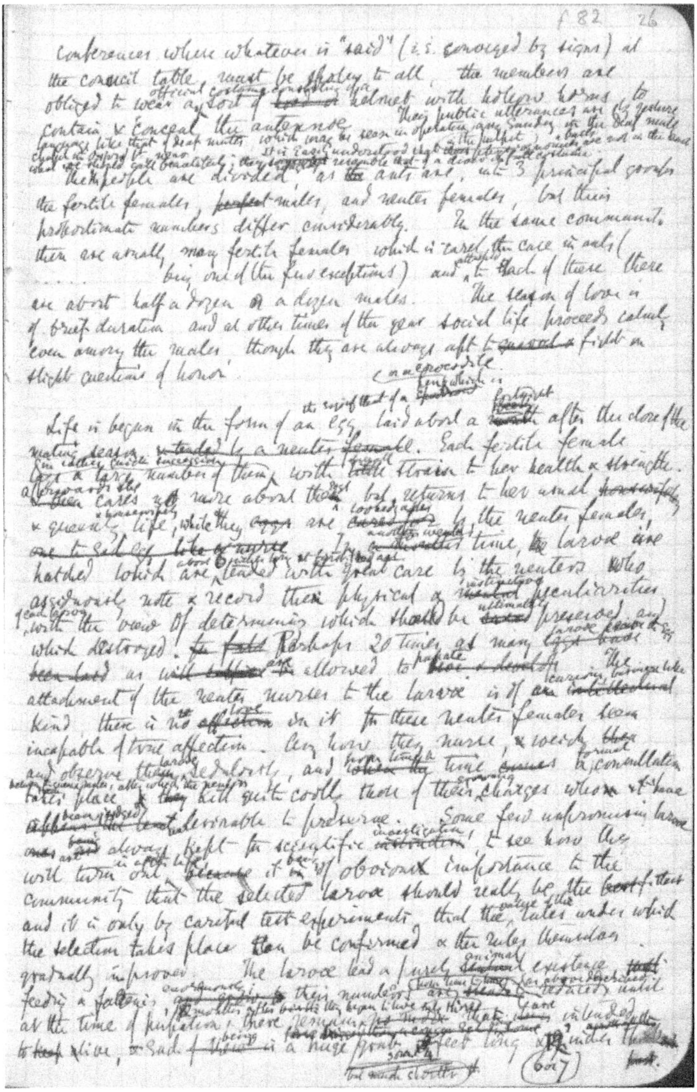

Figure 5.5: Page 26 of the Notebook.

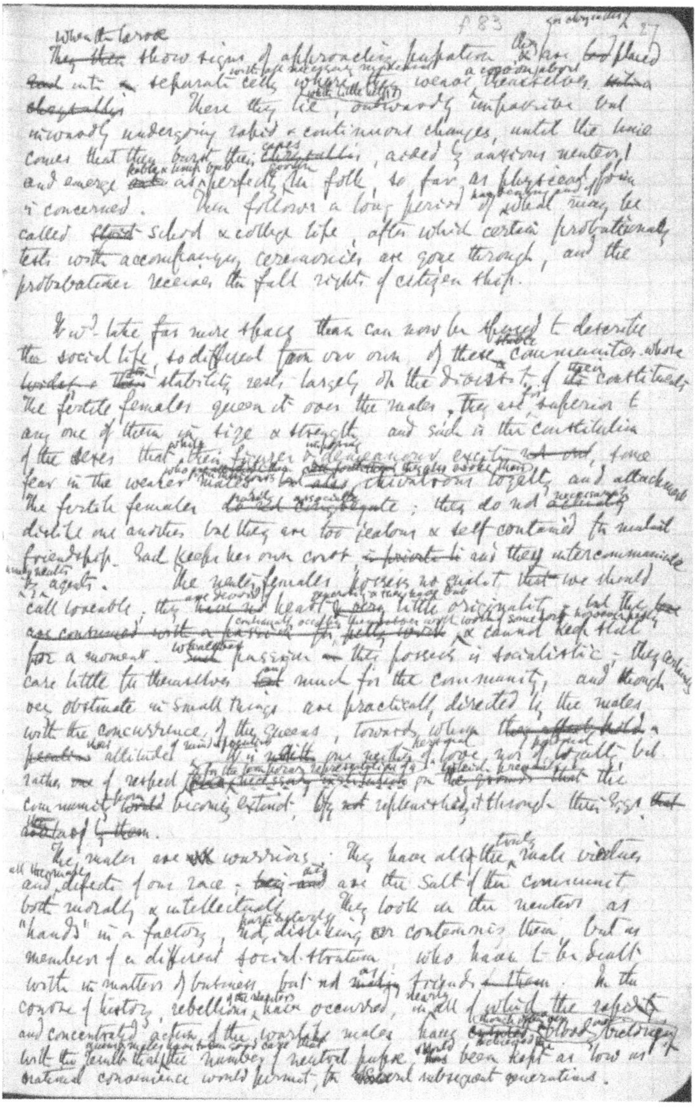

When the larvae show signs of approaching pupation they are placed into separate cells where they weave themselves a cocoon. There they lie, outwardly impassive but inwardly undergoing rapid & continuous changes, until the time comes that they burst their cases, aided by anxious neuters, and emerge as perfect as they will, so far as physical form is concerned. Then follows a long period of what may be called school & college life, after which certain probationary tests with accompanying ceremonies are gone through, and the probationer receives the full rights of citizenship.

It w^d take far more space than can now be spared to describe the social life, so different from our own, of these strange communities whose stability rests largely on the diversity of their constitution. The fertile females queen it over the males, they are superior to any one of them in size & strength and such is the constitution of the sexes that while their presence & demeanour excite fear in the weaker males, chivalrous loyalty and attachment. The fertile females ...; they do not ... dislike one another but they are too jealous & self contained for mutual friendship. Each keeps her own court and they intercommunicate mainly by agents. The neuter females possess no quality that we should call loveable, they are devoid of heart, very little originality, but they ... & cannot keep still for a moment. ... passion they possess is socialistic; they care little for themselves and much for the community, and though over obstinate in small things are practically directed by the males with the concurrence of the queens, towards whom their attitude is not one of love nor of loyalty but rather of respect ... the community would become extinct ...

The males are warriors. They have all the truly male virtues and defects of our race & are the salt of the community both morally & intellectually. They look on the neuters as "hands" in a factory, not disliking or contemning them, but as members of a different social stratum, who have to be dealt with in matters of business, but not as friends. In the course of history, rebellions have occurred, nearly all of which the rapid and concentrated action of the warlike males have ... bloody ... with the result that the number of neutral pupae has been kept as low as national convenience would permit, for several subsequent generations.

Figure 5.6: Page 27 of the Notebook.

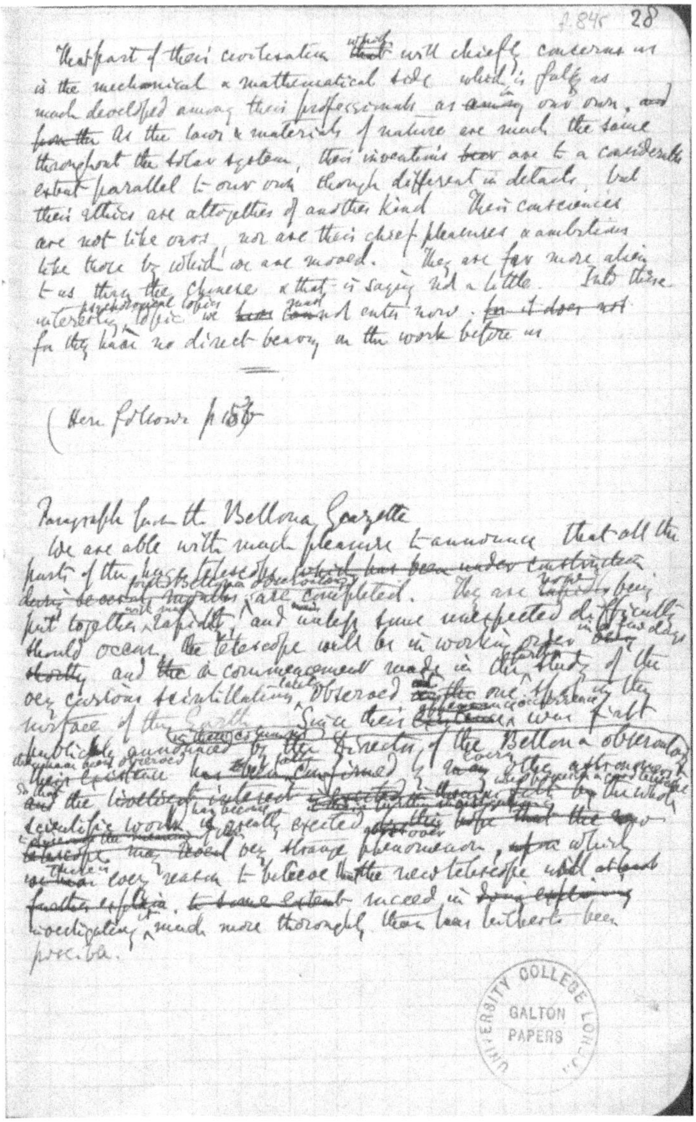

That part of their conversation which will chiefly concern us is the mechanical & mathematical side which is fully as much developed among their professionals as among our own, and As the laws & materials of nature are much the same throughout the solar system, their inventions are to a considerable extent parallel to our own though different in details, but their ethics are altogether of another kind. Their consciences are not like ours, nor are their chief pleasures & ambitions like those by which we are moved. They are far more alien to us than the Chinese & that is saying not a little. Into these psychological topics we need not enter now, for they have no direct bearing on the work before us

(Here follows p [illegible])

Paragraph from the Bellona Gazette

We are able with much pleasure to announce that all the parts of the large telescope of the Bellona Observatory are completed. They are now being put together with much rapidity, and unless some unexpected difficulty should occur, the telescope will be in working order in a few days and a commencement made in the study of the very curious scintillations lately observed on the surface of the Earth. Since their occurrence was first publicly announced by the Director of the Bellona observatory [illegible] confirmed by every other astronomer who possesses a good telescope, so that the liveliest interest has been excited [illegible] the whole scientific world [illegible] very strange phenomena, [illegible] there is every reason to believe the new telescope will succeed in investigating it much more thoroughly than has hitherto been possible.

Figure 5.7: Page 28 of the Notebook.

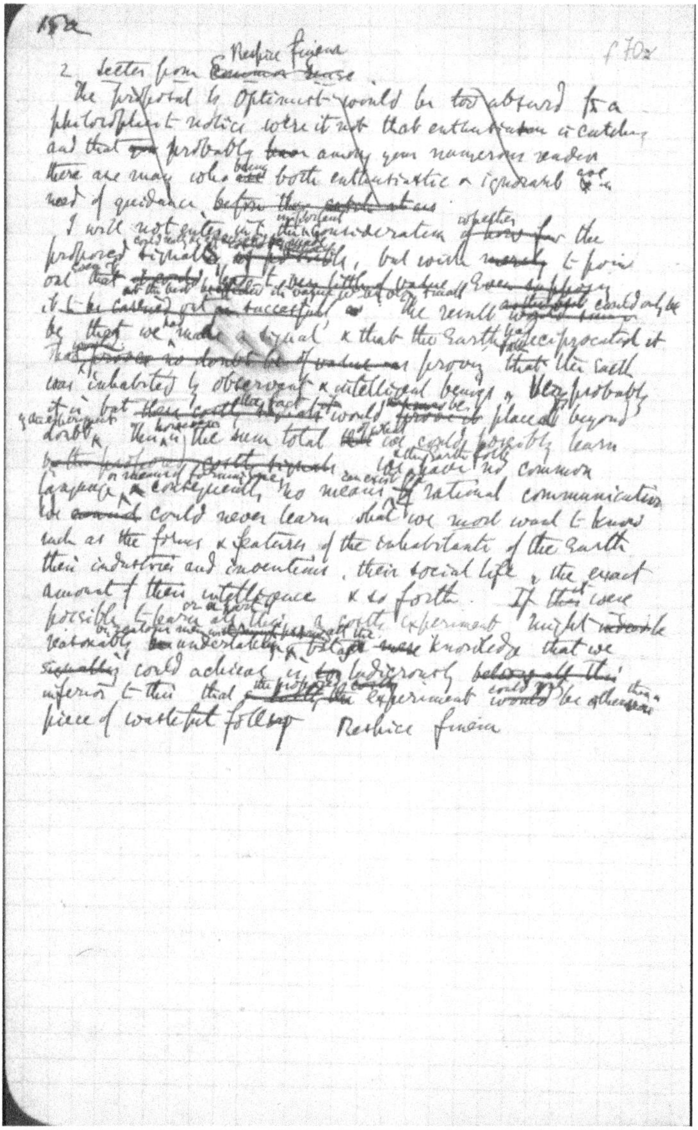

1892 f 70z

2 Letter from Common Sense Respice finem

The proposal to Optimist would be too absurd for a philosophical notice were it not that enthusiasm is catching and that probably among your numerous readers there are many who being both enthusiastic & ignorant are in need of guidance.

I will not enter into the consideration whether the proposed signals [illegible], but wish to point out that [illegible] even supposing it to be carried out successfully the result could only be that we made a signal & that the Earth people reciprocated it [illegible] proving that the earth was inhabited by observant & intelligent beings & very probably [illegible] would be placed beyond doubt. This however is the sum total we could possibly learn [illegible] no common language & consequently no means of rational communication we could never learn what we most want to know such as the forms & features of the inhabitants of the earth their industries and inventions, their social life & the exact amount of their intelligence & so forth. If it were possible to learn all this a costly experiment might reasonably be undertaken [illegible] knowledge that we could achieve is so ludicrously inferior to this that the proposed experiment could be [illegible] piece of wasteful folly. Respice finem

Figure 5.8: Page 15a of the Notebook, Part 1.

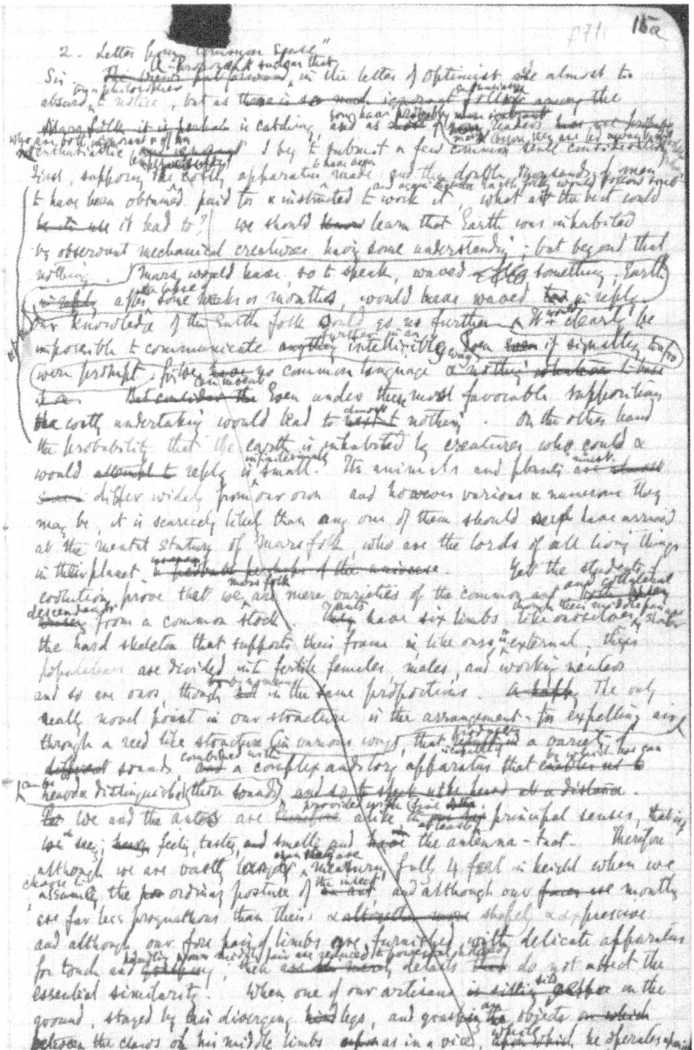

Figure 5.9: Page 15a of the Notebook, Part 2.

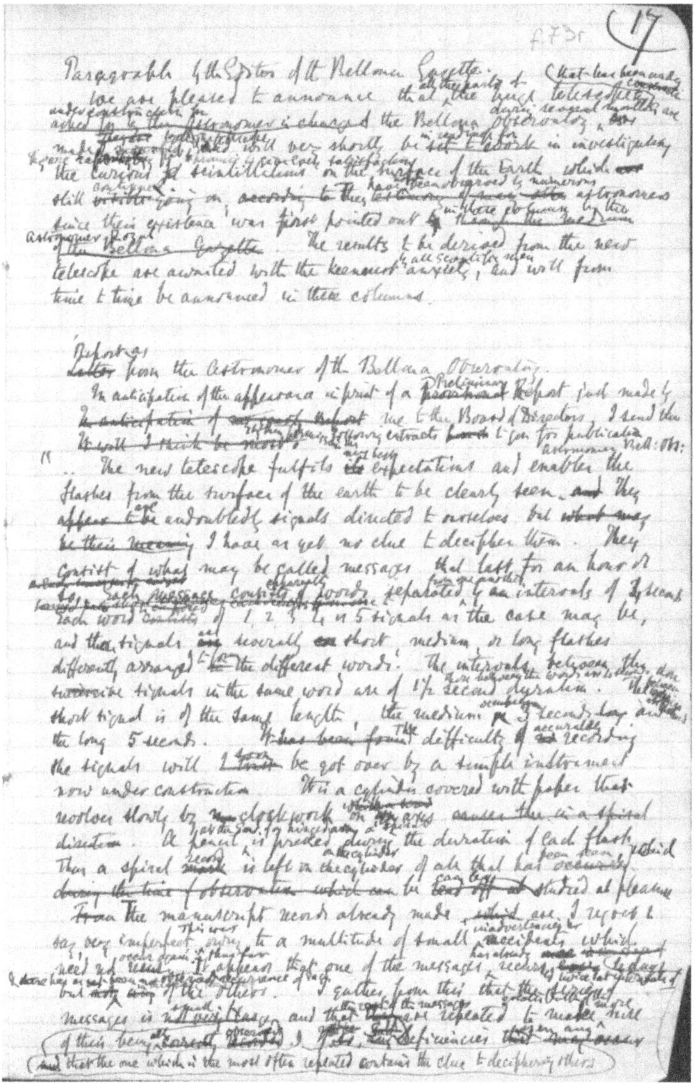

Figure 5.10: Page 17 of the Notebook.

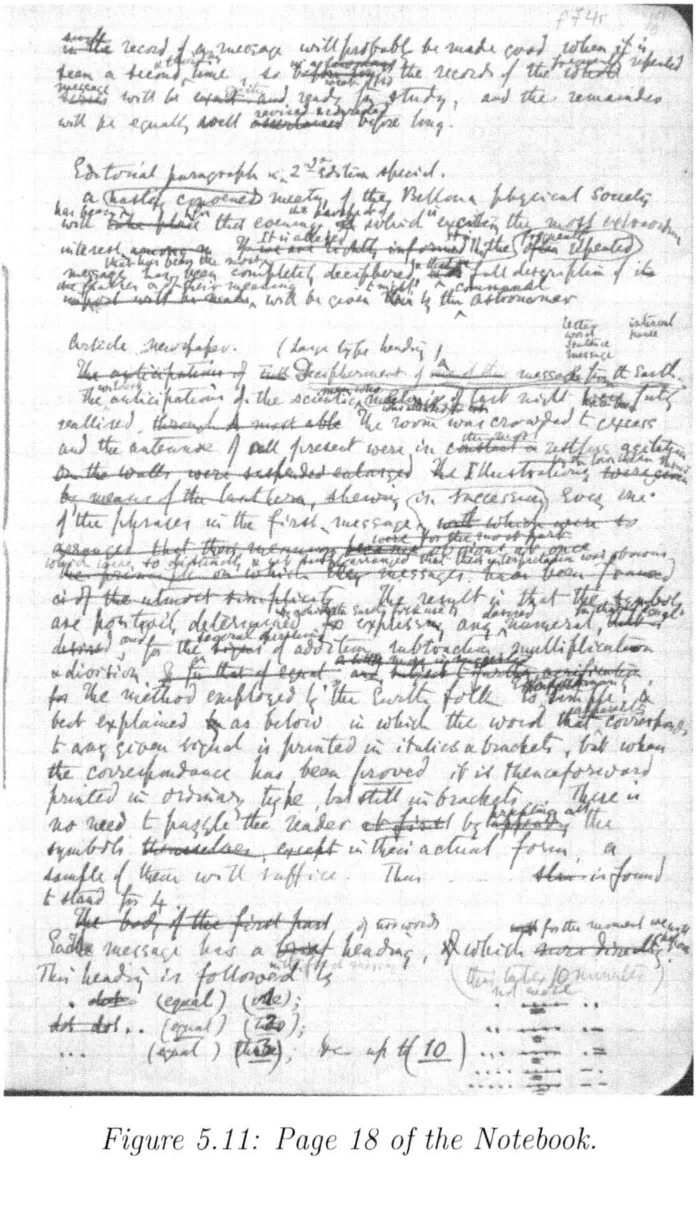
the record of any message will probably be made good when it is seen a second time, so that the record of the frequently repeated message will be exact and ready for study, and the remainder will be equally well revised before long.

Editorial paragraph in 2nd Edition special.

A hastily convened meeting of the Bellona Physical Society will take place this evening which excites the most extraordinary interest.

Article newspaper. (Large type heading)

The anticipation of the scientific world was fully realised. The room was crowded to excess and the attention of all present were in the utmost restless agitation. The Illustrations ... shewing in succession every one of the phrases in the first message ... The result is that the symbols are positively determined to express any numeral, ... for the several symbols of addition, subtraction, multiplication & division ... for the method employed by the Earth folk to ... is best explained as below in which the word that corresponds to any given symbol is printed in italics & brackets, but when the correspondence has been proved it is thenceforward printed in ordinary type, but still in brackets. There is no need to puzzle the reader by ... the symbols except in their actual form. A sample of them will suffice. Thus ... is found to stand for 4.

Each message has a heading, which ...

This heading is followed by

. (equal) (one);

.. (equal) (two);

... (equal) (three), &c up to (10)

Figure 5.11: Page 18 of the Notebook.

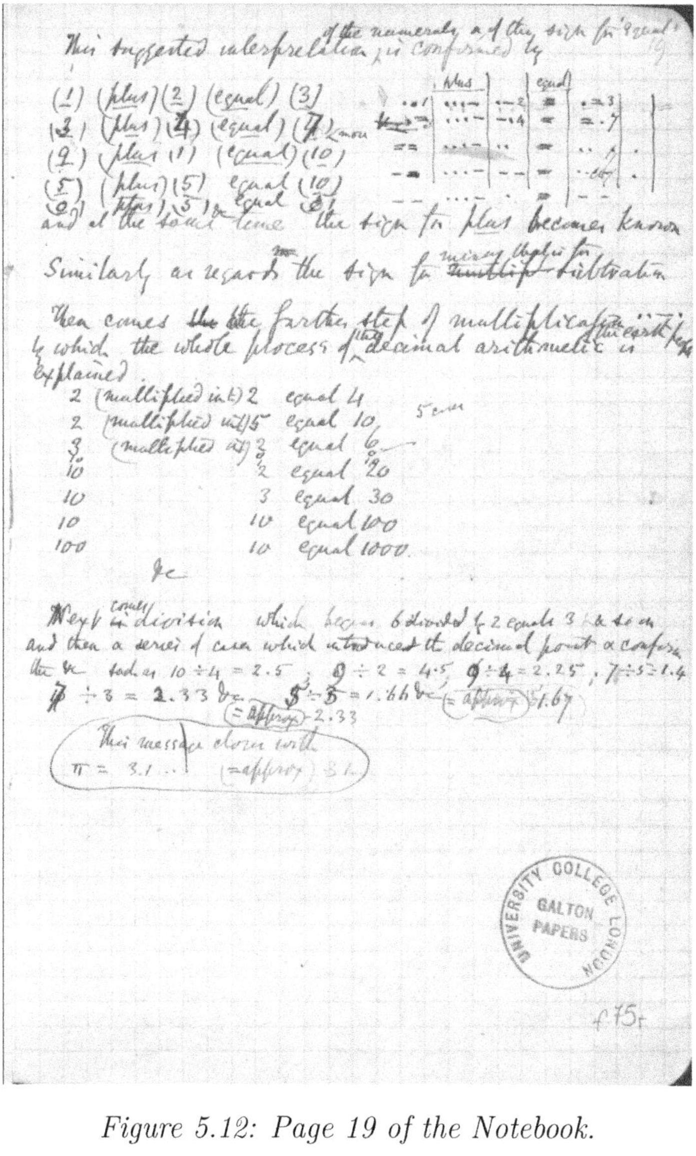

This suggested interpretation of the numerals and of the sign for 'equal' is confirmed by

(1) (plus) (2) (equal) (3)
(3) (plus) (4) (equal) (7) known
(9) (plus) (1) (equal) (10)
(5) (plus) (5) equal (10)

and at the same time the sign for plus becomes known

Similarly as regards the sign for minus (subtraction)

Then comes the further step of multiplication by which the whole process of the decimal arithmetic is explained

2 (multiplied into) 2 equal 4
2 (multiplied into) 5 equal 10
3 (multiplied into) 2 equal 6
10 2 equal 20
10 3 equal 30
10 10 equal 100
100 10 equal 1000
&c

Next comes division which begins 6 divided by 2 equals 3 & so on and then a series of cases which introduced the decimal point & confirm the &c such as 10 ÷ 4 = 2.5 ; 9 ÷ 2 = 4.5, 9 ÷ 4 = 2.25, 7 ÷ 5 = 1.4
7 ÷ 3 = 2.33 &c. 5 ÷ 3 = 1.66 &c (= approx 1.67)
(= approx) 2.33

This message closes with
π = 3.1 ... (= approx) 3.1

UNIVERSITY COLLEGE LONDON GALTON PAPERS

f 75r

Figure 5.12: Page 19 of the Notebook.

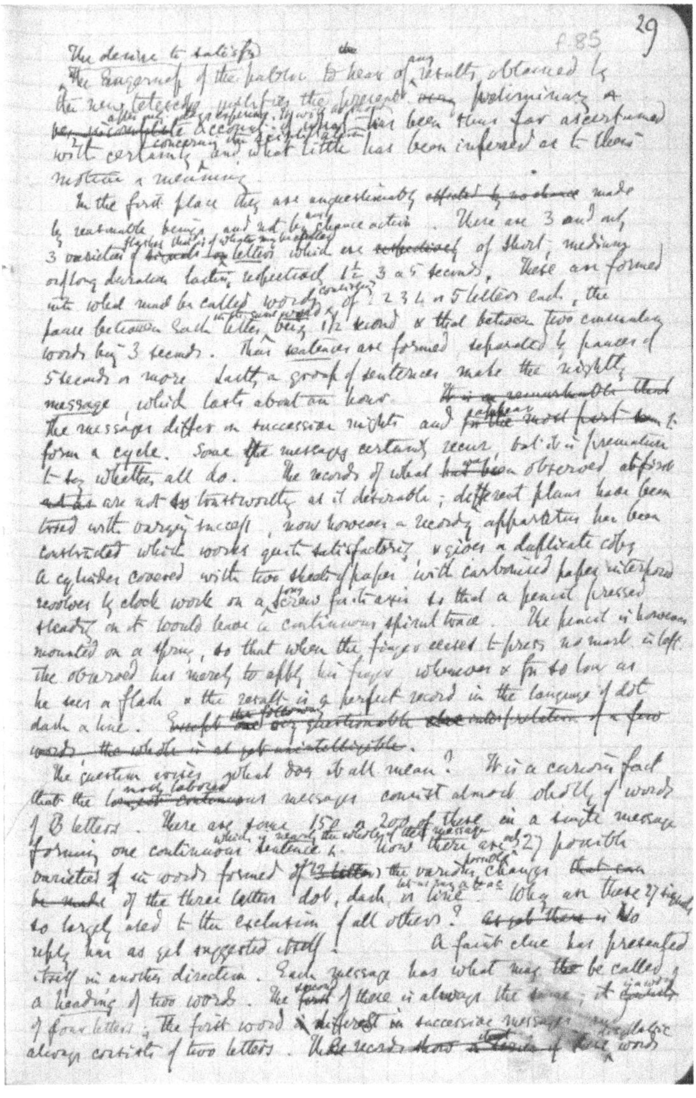

29

f.85

The desire to satisfy the
~~The~~ eagerness of the public to hear of any results obtained by the new telescope justifies the present ~~very~~ preliminary & ~~very incomplete~~ account [illegible] of what has been thus far ascertained with certainty and what little has been inferred as to their nature & meaning.

In the first place they are unquestionably ~~effected by rational~~ made by rational beings, and not by any chance action. There are 3 and only 3 varieties of [illegible] ~~letters~~ letters which are ~~respectively~~ of short, medium or long duration lasting respectively 1½, 3 & 5 seconds. These are formed into what must be called words consisting of 2 3 4 or 5 letters each, the pause between each letter being 1½ second & that between two consecutive words being 3 seconds. Then sentences are formed separated by pauses of 5 seconds or more. Lastly a group of sentences make the nightly message which lasts about an hour. ~~It is a remarkable that~~ The messages differ on successive nights and ~~for the most part~~ perhaps form a cycle. Some of the messages certainly recur, but it is premature to say whether all do. The records of what has been observed at first ~~and~~ are not as trustworthy as it desirable; different plans have been tried with varying success, now however a recording apparatus has been constructed which works quite satisfactorily & gives a duplicate copy. A cylinder covered with two sheets of paper with carbonized paper interposed revolves by clock work on a long screw for its axis so that a pencil pressed steadily on it would leave a continuous spiral trace. The pencil is however mounted on a spring, so that when the finger ceases to press no mark is left. The observer has merely to apply his finger whenever & for as long as he sees a flash & the result is a perfect record in the language of dot dash & line. ~~Except the following questionable interpretation of a few words the whole is as yet unintelligible.~~

The question arises what does it all mean? It is a curious fact that the ~~longest continuous~~ most labored messages consist almost wholly of words of 3 letters. There are some 150 or 200 of these in a single message forming one continuous sentence which nearly the whole of ~~the~~ message. Now there are only 27 possible varieties of such words formed ~~of 3 letters~~ by the various possible changes ~~that can be made~~ of the three letters dot, dash, or line taken three at a time. Why are these 27 signals so largely used to the exclusion of all others? ~~As yet there is~~ No reply has as yet suggested itself! A faint clue has presented itself in another direction. Each message has what may ~~the~~ be called a heading of two words. The ~~first~~ second of these is always the ~~same~~, it ~~[illegible]~~ [illegible] of four letters; the first word is different in successive messages and altogether always consists of two letters. The records ~~show~~ ~~[illegible]~~ of [illegible] words

Figure 5.13: Page 29 of the Notebook.

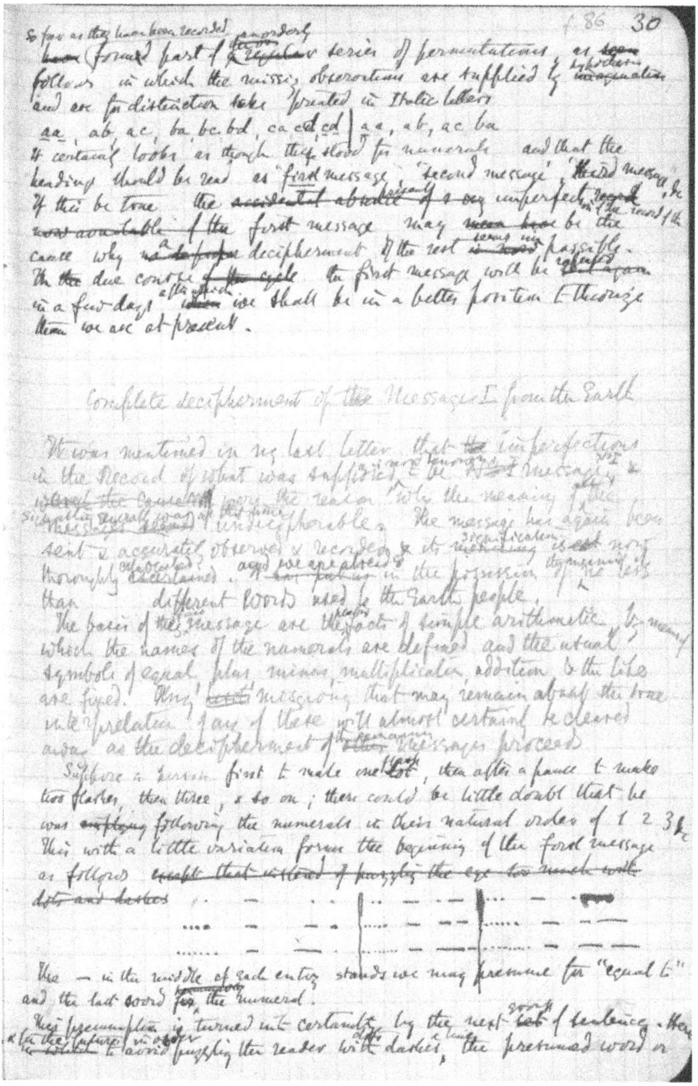
f. 86 30

so far as they have been recorded form part of a series of permutations, as follows in which the missing observations are supplied by hypothesis and are for distinction printed in Italic letters

aa, ab, ac, ba, bc, bd, ca, cd, cd | aa, ab, ac, ba

it certainly looks as though they stood for numerals and that the heading should be read as "first message", "second message", "third message" &c.

If this be true the imperfect record of the first message may be the cause why a decipherment of the rest seems impossible.

In due course the first message will be repeated in a few days after which we shall be in a better position to theorize than we are at present.

Complete decipherment of the Message I from the Earth

It was mentioned in my last letter that the imperfections in the Record of what was supposed to be the first message were the reason why the meaning of the messages seemed undecipherable. The message has again been sent & accurately observed & recorded & its signification is now thoroughly ascertained. and we are already in the possession of no less than different words used by the Earth people.

The basis of the message are the facts of simple arithmetic by means of which the names of the numerals are defined and the usual symbols of equal, plus, minus, multiplication, addition & the like are fixed. Any misgiving that may remain about the true interpretation of any of these will almost certainly be cleared away as the decipherment of the remaining messages proceeds.

Suppose a person first to make one flash, then after a pause to make two flashes, then three, & so on; there could be little doubt that he was following the numerals in their natural order of 1 2 3 &c.

This with a little variation forms the beginning of the first message as follows

The — in the middle of each entry stands we may presume for "equal to" and the last word for the numeral.

This presumption is turned into certainty by the next group of sentences. Here to avoid puzzling the reader with dots & dashes, the presumed word or

Figure 5.14: Page 30 of the Notebook.

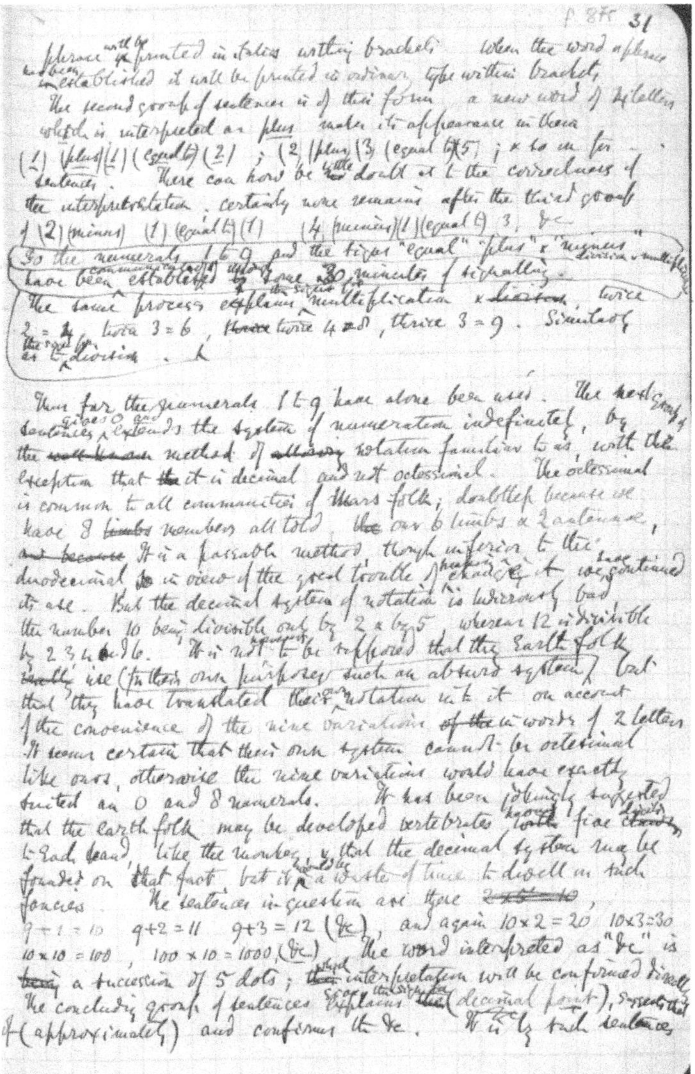

f. 875 31

phrase will be printed in italics within brackets. When the word or phrase has been established it will be printed in ordinary type within brackets.

The second group of sentences is of this form: a new word of 4 letters which is interpreted as plus makes its appearance in these (1) (plus) (1) (equal to) (2) ; (2) (plus) (3) (equal to) (5) ; & so on for ... sentences. There can now be little doubt as to the correctness of the interpretation. certainly none remains after the third group of (2) (minus) (1) (equal to) (1) (4) (minus) (1) (equal to) 3, &c.

So the numerals 1 to 9 and the signs "equal" "plus" & "minus" division & multiplication have been established communicated with by some 30 minutes of signalling.

The same process explains the signs for multiplication & division, twice 2 = 4, twice 3 = 6, twice 4 = 8, thrice 3 = 9. Similarly the sign for division.

Thus far the numerals 1 to 9 have alone been used. The next group of sentences gives 0 and extends the system of numeration indefinitely, by the method of notation familiar to us, with the exception that it is decimal and not octessimal. The octessimal is common to all communities of Mars folk; doubtless because we have 8 numbers all told, the our 6 limbs & 2 antennae. It is a passable method though inferior to the duodecimal in view of the great trouble of changing it we have continued its use. But the decimal system of notation is intrinsically bad the number 10 being divisible only by 2 & by 5, whereas 12 is divisible by 2 3 4 and 6. It is not supposed that the Earth folk use (for their own purposes) such an absurd system, but that they have translated their notation into it on account of the convenience of the nine variations in words of 2 letters. It seems certain that their own system cannot be octessimal like ours, otherwise the nine variations would have exactly suited an 0 and 8 numerals. It has been jokingly suggested that the Earth folk may be developed vertebrates having five digits to each hand, like the monkey, & that the decimal system may be founded on that fact but it would be a waste of time to dwell on such fancies. The sentences in question are these

9 + 1 = 10 9+2 = 11 9+3 = 12 (&c), and again 10×2 = 20 10×3=30 10 × 10 = 100, 100 × 10 = 1000 (&c). The word interpreted as "&c" is a succession of 5 dots; this interpretation will be confirmed directly. The concluding group of sentences explains the sign for (decimal point), suggests that of (approximately) and confirms the &c. It is by such sentences

Figure 5.15: Page 31 of the Notebook.

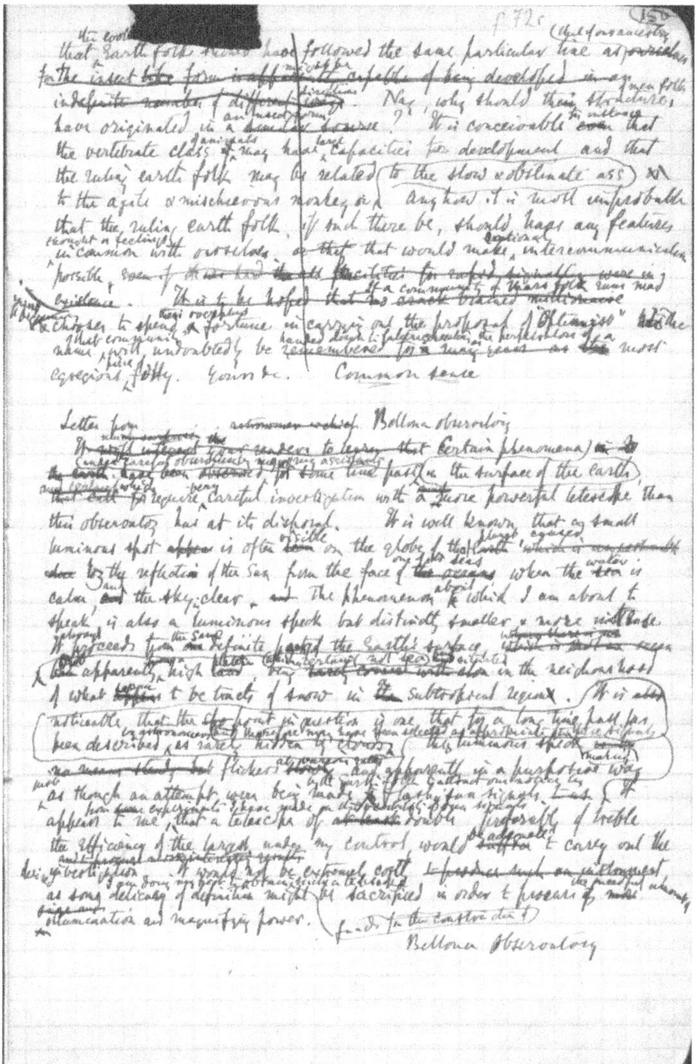

Figure 5.16: Page 15b of the Notebook.

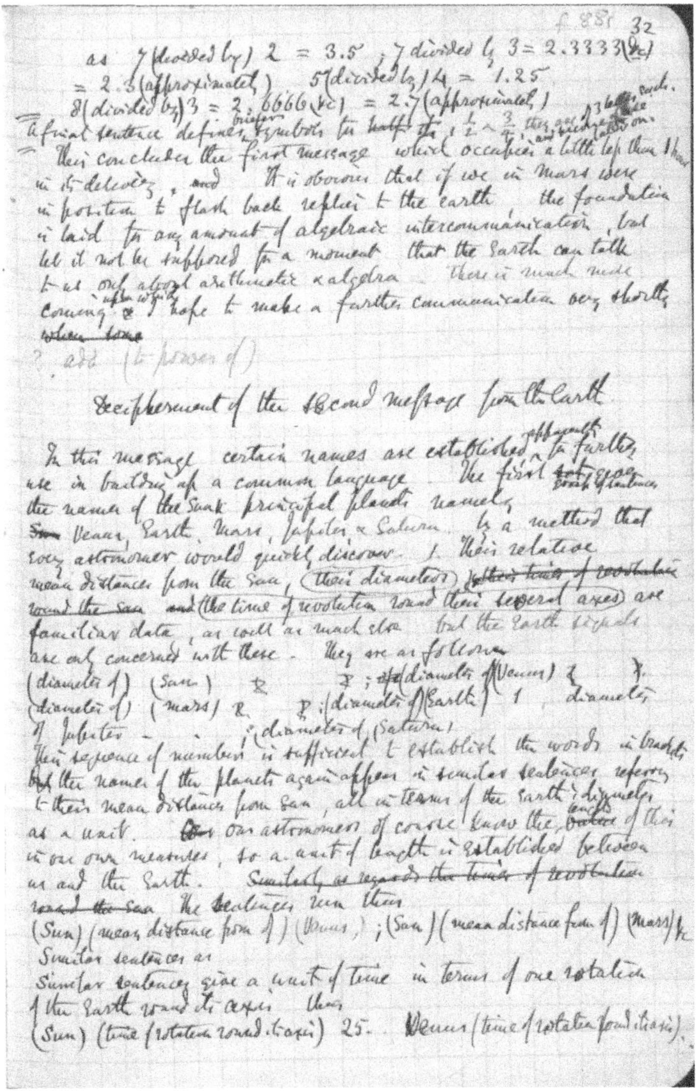

f. 88r 32

as 7 (divided by) 2 = 3.5 ; 7 divided by 3 = 2.3333 (&c) = 2.3 (approximately) 5 (divided by) 4 = 1.25
8 (divided by) 3 = 2.6666 (&c) = 2.7 (approximately)
The final sentence defines simpler symbols for half [illegible] $\frac{1}{2}$ & $\frac{3}{4}$, they are [illegible] and used [illegible] later on.
This concludes the first message which occupies a little less than 1 hour in its delivery, and It is obvious that if we in Mars were in position to flash back replies to the earth the foundation is laid for any amount of algebraic intercommunication, but let it not be supposed for a moment that the Earth can talk to us only about arithmetic & algebra. There is much more coming upon which I hope to make a further communication very shortly ~~when some~~
?, add (to power of)

Decipherment of the second message from the Earth

In this message certain names are established apparently for further use in building up a common language. The first ~~sets~~ group of sentences the names of the Sun & principal planets namely ~~Sun~~ Venus, Earth, Mars, Jupiter & Saturn by a method that every astronomer would quickly discover. The relative mean distances from the Sun, (their diameters) ~~their times of revolution round the Sun~~ ~~and~~ (the time of revolution round their several axes) are familiar data, as well as much else but the Earth signals are only concerned with these. They are as follows
(diameter of) (Sun) [illegible] [illegible] ; (diameter of)(Venus) [illegible] [illegible].
(diameter of) (Mars) [illegible] [illegible] ; (diameter of)(Earth) 1, diameter of Jupiter – ; diameter of (Saturn)
This sequence of numbers is sufficient to establish the words in brackets but the names of the planets again appear in similar sentences referring to their mean distances from Sun, all in terms of the earth's distance as a unit. ~~Our~~ Our astronomers of course know the ~~[illegible]~~ lengths of this in our own measures, so a unit of length is established between us and the Earth. ~~Similarly as regards the times of revolution round the Sun~~ The sentences run thus
(Sun) (mean distance from of) (Venus) ; (Sun) (mean distance from of) (Mars) [illegible]
Similar sentences as
Similar sentences give a unit of time in terms of one rotation of the Earth round its axis thus
(Sun) (time of rotation round its axis) 25. Venus (time of rotation round its axis).

Figure 5.17: Page 32 of the Notebook.

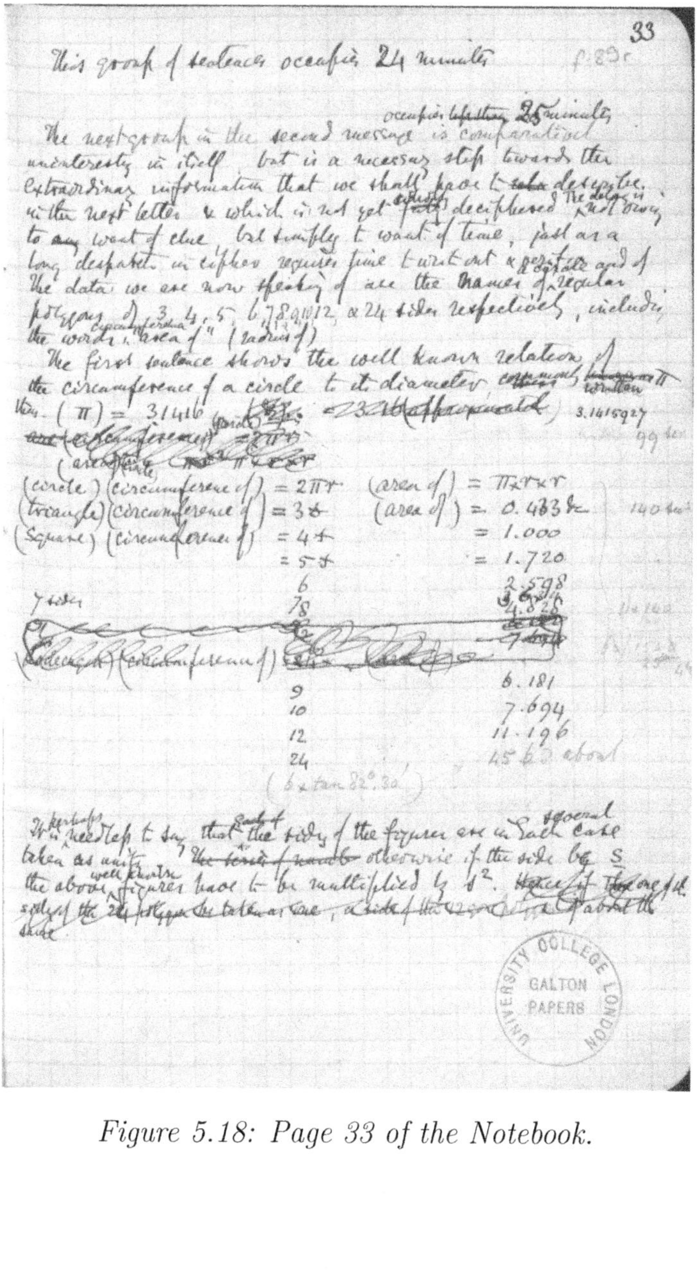

Figure 5.18: Page 33 of the Notebook.

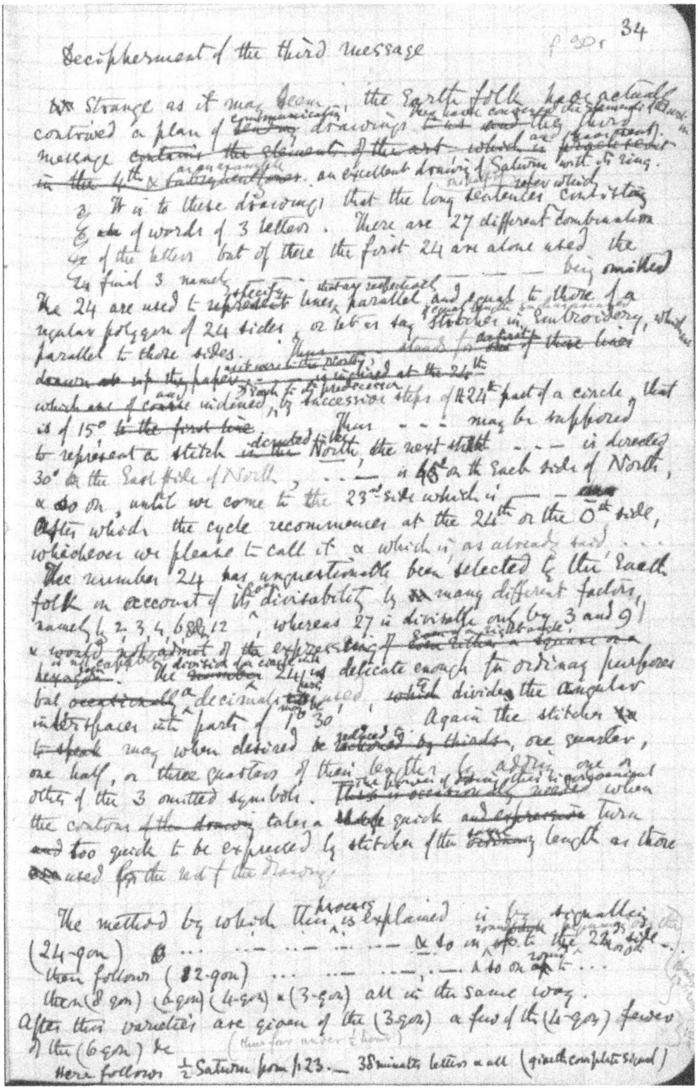
Decipherment of the third message f 30r 34

Strange as it may seem, the Earth folk have actually contrived a plan of communication drawings … the third message … an excellent drawing of Saturn with its ring.

It is to these drawings that the long sentences consisting of words of 3 letters. There are 27 different combinations of the letters but of these the first 24 are alone used, the final 3 namely … being omitted.

The 24 are used to represent lines, parallel and equal to those of a regular polygon of 24 sides, or let us say stitches in embroidery, which are parallel to those sides … which are of course inclined by successive steps of the 24th part of a circle, that is of 15°. Thus … may be supposed to represent a stitch directed to the North, the next … is directed 30° on the East side of North, … is 45° on the East side of North, & so on, until we come to the 23rd side which is … After which the cycle recommences at the 24th or the 0th side, whichever we please to call it … which is, as already said …

The number 24 has unquestionably been selected by the Earth folk on account of its divisibility by so many different factors, namely by 2, 3, 4, 6, 8 & 12, whereas 27 is divisible only by 3 and 9 … The 24 is delicate enough for ordinary purposes but a decimal is used, which divides the angular interspaces into parts of 1° 30'. Again the stitches may when desired be reduced to one quarter, one half, or three quarters of their length by adding one or other of the 3 omitted symbols … when the contour takes a quick turn too quick to be expressed by stitches of the length as those used for the rest of the drawing.

The method by which this process is explained is by signalling (24-gon) … & so on up to the 22nd side … then follows (12-gon) … & so on … then (8 gon) (6 gon) (4-gon) & (3-gon) all in the same way. After this varieties are given of the (3-gon) a few of the (4-gon) fewer of the (6 gon) &c (thus far under 2 hours)

Here follows ½ Saturn from p 23. — 38 minutes letters & all (gives the complete Saturn)

Figure 5.19: Page 34 of the Notebook.

Appendix A

Intelligible Signals Between Neighbouring Stars.

Considerable interest attaches itself to methods of communication which have been devised under the pressure of necessity, to take the place of speech and writing.[1] Many memoirs have, consequently, been written on such topics as the gesture language of savages, or that of deaf mutes, or on the alphabetical tappings of prisoners upon the walls that divide their solitary cells, or on Laura Bridgeman[2] and a few like her, who, though destitute of all other senses, have,

[1] Published in the *Fortnightly Review*, see Galton 1896a. This is a reworked version of the text in previous chapters, written from the point of view of Earth, with all the eugenic and other details about Martians omitted.

[2] Laura Dewey Lynn Bridgman (1829 –1889), a victim of scarlet fever.

nevertheless, been educated to a high level of accomplishment by touch alone. In most of these cases the method of instruction is by "trial and error." The pupil makes many guesses, the wrong ones are negatived by his teacher with a gesture of impatience, the right one is welcomed approvingly. But no help can be obtained from this method in the task I have set myself to perform. Signals have to be devised that are *intrinsically* intelligible, so that the messages may be deciphered by any intelligent man, or other creature, who has made nearly as much advance in pure and applied science as ourselves. It may seem at first sight almost impossible to do this, but it is quite otherwise, and the reader will probably feel surprised at the unexpected simplicity of this curious problem.

I may as well mention how it came into my thoughts. Some four years ago the planet Mars made a near approach to the earth, and presented a splendid spectacle at night. The possibility of exchanging visible signals with Mars was then discussed in the newspapers, apparently with the result that it was not altogether inconceivable that signals might be sent, though the difficulties of doing so would be enormous. Then the very different question arose of "cui bono?" to which there was a general response that nothing more could possibly be learnt on either side than that intelligent folk existed on the other planet, who were observant, mechanical, and capable of acting in unison upon large undertakings. For my part, I considered that limitation unjustified, and amused myself with thinking out the ground-plan of the present article. In the meantime the craze about Mars died away; the planet ceased to be particularly conspicuous, people grew tired of the topic, and the heated thoughts of many writers were cooled by copious douches of astronomical common sense. The subject having ceased to interest others, I laid up my ideas presumably for perpetuity, but an accident revived them. I was compelled last summer to spend a somewhat dreamy vacation, beginning with a course of hot baths at Wildbad, and its relaxing accompaniments (for the good effects of which I am truly grateful), when being unable to occupy myself otherwise than in a desultory way, I did so by developing my previous notions.

The simplest way of explaining my method is to suppose that Mars began to signal, to the wonderment of our astronomers, who sent descriptive letters to the newspapers from day to day, out of which the following imaginary extracts are taken:—

> 1. Astronomers in various observatories have been much excited of late by the sight of minute scintillations of light proceeding

from a single well-defined spot on the surface of Mars, and they are becoming greatly perplexed as to the significance of this strange phenomenon. It is hoped that the Director of the X. high level observatory, where the atmosphere is singularly transparent, which is favourably situated for now observing the spot in question, and which is furnished with a telescope peculiarly well suited for examining Mars, will soon be able to tell us something more about it. In the meantime it is well not to indulge too freely in wild speculation.

2. The Director of the X. observatory is, at last, strongly disposed to believe that the scintillations are purposive; that they are really intended as signals from the Mars-folk to the earth. He suspects that their signalling apparatus is not yet in working order, that adjustments are being verified, and that what we now see resembles the tuning of instruments before the opera begins. If the signals are produced as they seem to be, by an immense assemblage of large heliographs, the difficulty would be great in drilling the multitude of operators engaged in working them simultaneously.

3. The scintillations from Mars show more firmness and power, but the signalling is still in the earlier stage of preliminary trials. Enough has, however, been seen to show that three and only three different signals are employed, differing in their lengths, and which for brevity may be called *dot*, *dash*, and *line*. The dot lasts $1\frac{1}{4}$ seconds, the dash $2\frac{1}{2}$, and the line 5 seconds; consequently the mean length of a signal is a trifle under 3 seconds. There have been a few well marked successions of "dot, dash, line", "dot, dash, line," in which the interval between the several letters, so to speak, is $1\frac{1}{2}$ seconds; those between words, one of which is here represented by a short bar, are 3 seconds; those between paragraphs are 6 seconds. This may be accepted as a good estimate of the future speed of signalling, though, of course, the exigencies of experience may show that a slower rate will be needed, or, again, the drill may hereafter be so smartly performed, that the rate will be increased. As there are three varieties of signal, the total number of different words of one letter is 3; of two letters, 9; of three letters, 27; of four letters, 81; of five let-

ters, 243, and so on. Also the average times occupied in signalling these words, including the 3 seconds' pause at the end of each, are 6, 10, 15, 20 and 24 seconds respectively. Whatever the Marsfolk may have to say must be briefly expressed, and it seems incredible under these conditions that anything could be communicated by them to us which shall be intelligible and of value. Some persons are disposed to ascribe this immense undertaking to the caprice of a mad millionaire in Mars, or rather to a mad billionaire. There have been instances in the past history of our earth of many gigantic follies, without counting the traditional Tower of Babel.

A recording apparatus is now constructed for our use here, which acts well. A long strip of telegraph paper is slowly drawn by clockwork under a hinged pencil on which the observer rests his finger. When a flash is on, he presses with his finger and the pencil leaves a mark; when the flash is off, he ceases to press, a spring lifts the pencil, and a blank is left on the travelling slip of paper.

4. The signals have improved considerably in regularity and power, and occasional

sequences of them have been gone through in a masterly way. So the drilling of the operators appears to be nearly complete, and we may expect soon to see what the system is intended to show. The phenomenon is most extraordinary. If it be effected through the money of a mad millionaire, he must have had the sense to subsidise an uncommonly intelligent director of works.

5. A most eventful night has been passed at the X. observatory. At first the sky was hazy and partly clouded, so Mars was, at the best, but imperfectly seen, and was often quite invisible; then, at half-past nine, all cloudiness disappeared, and the flashes were observed to be proceeding from Mars with greater power and precision than ever before. The whole assemblage of their heliographs must have been simultaneously at work, and the drill was excellent. The signalling continued off and on for more than three hours. The recorder being kept at work the whole time, every signal then made is preserved in a permanent form, of course including occasional mistakes. The records are as yet totally unintelligible, possibly owing to the loss of the first part of the com-

munication, which may have contained the key to what followed. It is noticeable that during the last two hours the signals consisted almost wholly of three-letter words; in the earlier part there was a preponderance of two-letter words, some of four and of five letters, but none of three.

6. A large typed telegraphic dispatch appeared in all the evening newspapers—

COMPLETE DECIPHERMENT OF THE FIRST PART OF THE MESSAGE FROM MARS. Full particulars tomorrow.

(Signed) Director of the X. Observatory.

7. The evening was serene, and the whole of the night continued to be beautifully clear. The experiences of previous days enabled every preparation to be made for the expected event. And it came. First there was a succession of "lines" with intervening pauses, evidently as a note of preparation, and then after a longer pause the message began with the accompanying sentence, which occupied less than six minutes in transmission.

No. of dots		is equal to	Symbols for numerals
1	.	-	. .
2	. .	-	. -
3	. . .	-	. —
4	. . . .	-	- .
5	. . . . .	-	- -
6	. . . . . .	-	- —
7	. . . .	-	— .
8	. . . .	-	. . — -
9	. . . .	-	. . . .
10	. . . .	-	. . . -
&c.	. . . .	-	. . . .

The headings and the column on the left, did not form part of the signalling, but are introduced for the convenience of the reader. The message is divided into three sub-divisions by means of pauses. Let us consider the first of these, in which there are seven lines. Every line begins with one or more dots; then follows a dash; and then a word of two letters. There is one dot at the beginning of the first line, two at that of the next, and so on regularly up to the seventh. The symbols at the end of the successive lines are those of the successive combinations of *dot*, *dash*, and *line*, taken in order up to the seventh; the eighth which is — -, and the ninth, which is — —, are not used. The arrangement suggests that the dash means "is equal to," and that the symbols are those of numerals, corresponding to the number of dots at the beginning of the line. So we should read the message as (one dot) (is equal to) 1; (two dots) (are equal to) 2, and so on. Accepting this interpretation provisionally, we see in the second subdivision that the symbols for 8, 9, and 10 are respectively represented by two words, thus 1?, 11, 12. The symbol here expressed by ? is the first of the two omissions mentioned above; it stands presumably for 0. This would show that the Mars-folk have not used a decimal system of notation as we do, but one that has 8 for its basis. With much hesitation, we may lastly suppose the four dots at the beginning and end of the line that forms the last subdivision, to mean "&c." so that line should read, &c. = &c.[3]

These provisional hypotheses are so amply confirmed by the next messages that ordinary figures will be used in place of the actual signals, and our own decimal notation will be employed, having first translated the Mars notation into it. Hereafter, Italic numerals and letters will signify suggested interpretations; after these have been confirmed and established, Roman ones will be substituted.

The second message consists of five lines:–
1 plus 1 (equal to) 2; 1 plus 2 (equal to) 3; 2 plus 3 (equal to) 5; 2 plus 5 (equal to) 7; 3 plus 3 (equal to) 6.

This goes a long way towards verifying the numerals, and it suggests the symbol for plus.

The third message is of a similar form, except that minus is substituted for plus, It adds so much confirmation to what has

[3] Galton must be indicating by the spacing that there are longer gaps between these dots, otherwise they could be confused with those meaning the numeral 4.

gone before that Italics need not be used for the simple numerals 1 to 7, nor for the words "equal to," "plus," and "minus." Each of these two messages occupied about 6 minutes.

Multiplication follows, by which the supposed system of notation with 8 for its basis is confirmed, and the symbol for 0 is established. The signals were, 2 (multiplied into) 2 (is equal to) 4; 2 (multiplied into) 3 (is equal to) 6. Then, after a double pause, 2 (multiplied into) 0 (is equal to) 0; 3 (multiplied into) 0 (is equal to) 0. This was followed by a series of higher multiples, such as we, writing in the decimal notation, might phrase as follows (the figures really used being different and accordant with a notation having 8 for its basis): 5 x 2 = 10; 10 x 10 = 100; 10 x 100 = 1000; 10 x 2 = 20; 10 x 3 = 30; 10 x 9 = 90; 7 x 3 = 21; 5 x 9 = 45; 9 x 9 = 81. Brackets were also expressed by 2 x 2 + 1 = 5; 2 x (2 + 1) = 6, and by two other messages of the same kind; the symbol for each bracket being a "line." The whole of this multiplication message occupied 16 minutes.

Division was then reached, by which the

symbol which corresponds to our "decimal" point was established, and the meaning of "&c." was confirmed. The message is of this form: 6 (divided by) 3 = 2; 12 (divided by) 4 = 3. Then, 5 (divided by) 2 = 2.5; 7 (divided 4) + = 1.75; 10 (divided by) 3 = 3.333, &c.

The whole of the division message occupied 15 minutes. Consequently the entire time spent thus far in actual signalling was 49 minutes. Adding about 10 minutes for intervening pauses, and another 15 for a long ... pause at the close, this portion of the communication occupied one hour and a quarter. The records of the previous night agreed in form with these, but the examples chosen for the arithmetical operations differed. A superabundance of evidence is, therefore, already to hand to prove the justice of the interpretations.

It will be observed that the seven numerals, 1 to 7, the 0, and the equivalent to our decimal point, exactly use up the nine words of two letters each. It is, therefore, conceivable that 8 may have been taken by the Mars-folk as the basis of their notation in these signals, on this account alone, and not because it is the system in ordinary use by them. A clever little girl who has helped us much by her quick guesses, intreats me to add her own peculiar view, which is that the Mars-folk are nothing more than highly developed ants, who count up to 8 by their 6 limbs and 2 antennae, as our forefathers counted up to 10 on their fingers. But enough of this.

There are a few apparent imperfections in the ensuing records, so I shall be glad of the experience of a third night, to revise thoroughly what has been already registered, and will, therefore, close my narrative for the present.

8. After the pause of fifteen minutes mentioned above, presumably to give time to the operators to readjust their instruments and to rest, the signals recommenced with the purpose of determining symbols to express the sun and the five principal planets. This was effected by three series of figures relating successively to nine distances from the sun, to their respective radii, and to times of rotation on their axes. The units of length were such that the earth's mean distance was taken as 100 in the first series,

and her diameter as 100 in the second series; similarly her time of diurnal rotation was taken as 100 in the third series. Doubtless the Mars-folk thought that the values under those forms would suggest their meanings the more readily to terrestrial astronomers. I give the messages in a compressed form, thus:— Sun (mean distance from) Sun (equal) 0; Venus (mean distance from) Sun (equal) 72; Earth (mean distance from) Sun (equal) 100; Mars, 153; Jupiter, 520; Saturn, 954.

Similarly, as regards the radii of the several planets: — Sun (radius of), 11,164; Venus, 97; Earth, 100; Mars, 53; Jupiter, 1,127; Saturn, 1004.

Here, however, either "diameter", or "circumference" would suit the context, as well as "radius." The assumed interpretation is confirmed later on, where the word radius is determined through a different connection. Another table of a similar kind refers to the relative periods of revolution on their respective axes.

Very little time was occupied in deciphering the above, as our whole staff were simultaneously engaged upon the records, all of whom were more or less familiar with these sequences of figures. When once the interpretation had been suggested, its truth was quickly seen to be beyond doubt, it being incredible that any other series of values should exist for which the above sequences might be mistaken. This astronomical message occupied twenty-five minutes and was accompanied and followed by a total pause of ten more.

9. Let it not be supposed that the value of the last and of the present message is confined to their intrinsic interests, for they are intended to introduce a descriptive method of a most unexpected and far-reaching character.

The signals recommenced with the series of figures which is perhaps the most familiar of all to mathematicians and astronomers, namely that which expresses the relation of the circumference of a circle to its diameter, or to double its radius. We always symbolise that relation by the Greek letter π, and usually symbolise the radius by r. The signals were — π (equal to) 3.1415592, &c. (circle) (perimeter of) (equal to) 2 (multiplied into) π (multiplied into) r.

There cannot be a doubt as to the second pair of these signals meaning π and r and of the first pair meaning "circle" and "perimeter"; which is soon explained. In the first place, these signals are followed by (circle) (area of) (equal to) π (multiplied into) r (multiplied into) r, which is a most familiar formula, and by determining both "circle" and r, it establishes "perimeter" and "π" After this came a series of signals for establishing eight new words, which seeming, at first sight to be little worth the trouble taken about them, are in reality important data. They are the names of the following regular polygons, as determined by their perimeters in one series and by their areas in another: namely, an equilateral triangle, a square, a pentagon, hexagon, octagon, dodecagon, and one with twenty-four sides. The nomenclature of the polygons is contrived to suggest their proper interpretations, by prefacing their names with the number that expresses the number of their respective sides. The first series runs (3-gon) (perimeter) (equal to) 3; (4-gon) (perimeter) (equal to) 4, and so on. The second series is (3-gon) (area) (equal to) 4.33; (4-gon) (area) (equal to) 1.00; (5-gon) (area) (equal to) 1.72, and so on. The sequence of the first series is obvious; that of the second is fairly well known, otherwise it can be easily calculated. Of course the sides are in each case taken as equal to 1. The time occupied in the actual signalling of the two series was twenty-five minutes, or including short pauses in the middle and a longer one at the end, thirty-five minutes.

10. We now reach the threshold of the final and most marvellous stage, namely that of effective picture-writing in outlines by means of series of words of three letters. It will be shown how names of three letters are assigned to each of the 24 sides of a regular 24-gon, which are of course of the same length and are inclined to the same line (let us say to the north and south line) by successive increments of 15 degrees (the 360° into which we usually divide the circle, when divided by 24 being equal to 15°). Thus, the left-hand side of the 24-gon has a slope of 0, or of 360°, whichever we please to call it; the adjacent side, proceeding upwards, has one of 3°; the next, one of 45°, and so on all round the compass. They would be the same in their directions as the so-called "rhumbs" of

a mariner's compass, if sailors divided their cards into 24 and not into 32 "points," If we take every second side of the 24-gon, and bring them together, they form a 12-gon. If we take every third side, the result will be an octagon; similarly for the hexagon and equilateral triangle. The symbols for the 24 sides are, as mentioned already, words of three letters; now there are 27 such words: consequently 3 remain over; one of these was used for "-gon," and another is found to be employed for "picture-writing," because it precedes every communication of the kind and is accompanied by a register number, to admit, as we may suppose, of each message being hereafter identifiable. The message by which this information is conveyed is of the following form, in which, for the convenience of the reader, the directions of the several sides are given in degrees of arc of our scale, though the 24 letters, a, b, c, &c., up to x, would more closely represent the actual signals.

It began by (picture formula), followed by a short pause; then—

(Picture formula) (24-gon) (equal to) 0°,

15°, 45°, &c., to 345°

(Picture formula) (12-gon) (equal to) 0°, 45°, 90°, &c., to 315°,

and so on all through the series. We may look on the picture formula as expressing the directions of each consecutive stitch in a piece of embroidery, those stitches being all of equal length.

There was some delay in puzzling out the above interpretation; it was first discovered by the young lady mentioned above, who is more successful than most of her companions in guessing charades and at such like games.

Further messages show that both the length of the stitch and its inclination may be specified more delicately by the help of decimals. Thus let j be the symbol for a stitch in any given direction, then $0.5 \times j$ means at half-length stitch in the direction j. A series of 4 triangles were signalled to explain this, in which the angles corresponded exactly with certain of the rhumbs, while the sides had to be expressed with decimals. Similarly as to the decimal division of the direction between rhumbs; in the first instance the pentagon was described, and then a series of four triangles, in which the sides were integral and the angles decimal. Short stitches are useful where the contour makes a sharp turn; minuteness of direction is sometimes wanted for the long lines in diagrams, but never for the short lines. Decimal directions are distinguished by brackets, thus $(0.3j)$ It will be recollected that the symbols for brackets, which are simply "lines," were determined during the multiplication message. The actual signalling of all the information described in this and the preceding letter occupied one hour and ten minutes, which was increased to an hour and a half by the pauses during its transmission and at its close.

11. A rapid retrospect may now be taken of what has been accomplished by less than two-and-a-half hours of actual signalling, together with pauses occupying a little less than one hour, making a total of three-and-a-half hours altogether. We have been made to completely understand the numerical notation of the Marsfolk, including their equivalent to our decimal point, and we have learnt the following twenty-nine words:—Area, bra-

ckets, circle, circumference, distance from, divided by, dodecagon, earth, equal to, etcetera, hexagon), Jupiter, Mars, minus, multiplied into, octagon, " ",[4] pentagon, perimeter of, picture-formula, radius, rhumb, Saturn, square, sun, twelve-sided regular polygon, triangle, equilateral triangle, Venus. We have also learnt how to draw any triangle, and implicitly how to draw any polygon, regular or irregular, from a picture-formula.

We now proceed to the ordinary picture-formulae, of which nine have been received in the six nights during which the signals have been recorded. The power of the method is easily seen by drawing any outline with dots at equal distances apart, and counting those dots. A dozen or fifteen are quite sufficient to indicate a figure, or a letter, or other simple object, and as each dot occupies at quarter of a minute to transmit, as many as 210 can be sent in an hour. A considerable assistance to ensuring the accuracy of the method is given by selecting convenient points of reference in the drawing, which we may call A, B, C, &c., and by giving the distance of each of them from one or more

[4] Galton actually has " ," but this is confusing.

of the others. This divides the drawing into stages, any one of which may be faulty without prejudice to the rest. It also enables detached parts to be drawn, commencing at one of the letters as a point of departure and ending at another. The points of reference are signalled thus:—A (distance to) B 42j; B (distance to) C 36d, and so on. The sign for "distance to" was determined in the letter No. 8.

The first of the pictures selected for decipherment was decided by the odd phrase (picture-formula) 0.5 (Saturn). It proved to be a beautiful representation of *one half* of Saturn and his ring. The other half, being symmetrical, did not need to be signalled. Only 105 "stitches" were employed. Another picture headed "Earth" proved to be a view of the American continent. 52 stitches sufficed for South America; but 88 were used for North America on account of the indentations of its shores; moreover, 16 of these were fractional stitches. A very good map was given of the solar system at the present date, so far as concerns the positions of the five principal planets about the sun. I must not at present speak of the do-

> mestic and sociological drawings, of which a new one is received every night, and the question whether or no the Mars-folk are glorified ants must remain for a short time longer in abeyance.

It is needless to continue in the same strain. I should say that the elements of the art of drawing outlines from written formulae that admit even of being telegraphed, was explained by me in a Friday Evening lecture, on the *Just Perceptible Difference*, at the Royal Institution in 1893.[5] Many illustrations of the method were then exhibited, one of which appears in the printed report. A large drawing of a Greek head had been made and formularised, then the formula was translated into dots upon paper, on the same large scale; rings were painted round the dots, and, lastly, the original and the copy were reduced by a photo-process to three different sizes. These form the printed illustrations. There were 271 dots, or rather rings, in this very effective picture, which contained the contour of the face, the sweep of the hair, the eyelids, and eyebrows.

It would be easy to enlarge the above vocabulary. Thus water and the metals could be defined by their relative specific gravities and other physical

5 Galton 1893.

properties; colours by diagrams of the prism and of the rainbow. Units of length and time have been already determined by the diameter of any given planet and the time of rotation on its axis; that of weight on the surface of any named planet could be determined also; and picture-writing would extend the list of named objects indefinitely. But substantives alone cannot form a language; the symbols for other parts of speech must be explained by pictures, those for the past, present, and future tenses by pictures of objects in motion.

It would be tedious, and is unnecessary to elaborate further, for it must be already evident to the reader that a small fraction of the care and thought bestowed, say, on the decipherment of hieroglyphics, would suffice to place the inhabitants of neighbouring stars in intelligible communication if they were both as far advanced in science and arts as the civilised nations of the earth at the present time. In short, that an efficient inter-stellar language admits of being established under those conditions, between stars that are sufficiently near together for signalling purposes.

FRANCIS GALTON

Appendix B

Signals available to men who are adrift on wrecks at sea.

TO THE EDITOR OF THE TIMES.[1] Sir —In *The Times* of to-day (Thursday) I have read with deep interest the fearful sufferings endured by a crew who were drifting about the Atlantic upon the wreck of their vessel. There is the old sad story repeated afresh by them, how, after days of anxious watching, first one vessel and then another were seen to approach hopefully, and then how each vessel, like its predecessor, passed by without noticing the low waterlogged wreck in which the sufferers were huddled, almost level with the sea, in the far distance. A distressed crew has little means of rigging up an object of suffi-

[1] Galton 1856a.

cient size to attract the attention of distant ships; but there is one signal, which is often a very practicable one and which seems well worthy of a sailor's notice. I do not for a moment suggest its use to the exclusion of any other methods, but only as a valuable addition to them; and, as the means for making it are simple and accessible, I should think no sailor or passenger should forget them, who, in the moment of impending disaster, makes a hasty rush down below deck to secure such light objects as may appear likely to be of service to him when adrift on a boat, raft, or wreck upon the wide ocean.

All that is wanted is a common looking-glass, even of the smallest size—a broken bit as large as two half-crowns will do—and with this he should glitter the rays of the sun towards the ship whose attention he wishes to attract. Even at a distance of ten miles the glitter from a looking-glass no larger than the mouth of a teacup appears as a radiant and glistering star, and would at once cause many eyes on board ship to be attentively directed upon it. It is a matter of some nicety to direct the glitter from a looking glass either steadily or accurately; and, as a sort of guide to the degree of accuracy required, I may remark that if such a thing were possible as that a man could actually see the glitter of the looking-glass in his hand against the blue vault of the sky, just as he may see it against the walls or ceiling of his room, that it would in all cases appear to him to be (within a most trivial degree of difference) of precisely the same size and shape as the sun itself, though excessively inferior in brightness.

The plan I use for directing the glitter with a just aim is to cut a small hole with a pocket knife in the middle of the board, or, it may be, of thin zinc plate, which forms the back of the looking-glass, and also to scratch away the quicksilver from below it, so as to leave a little round space of clear transparent glass as an eye-hole. Looking through this hole, I direct the centre of the glitter as truly as possible by watching the play of its edge upon some object that may happen to lie on one side or another of a line between the eye and the person I signal to. Thus, if a boat was being rowed in a direction somewhere towards a ship, a man sitting low down in the stern could direct the glitter of his looking glass by watching its play upon the bows of the boat at the moment when he could just catch sight of the ship over them. If a looking glass be used without first cutting a hole in its back in the way I have mentioned it is necessary to hold it close up under the eye, and to make more careful allowance for the height of the eye above it than a person who has not had a good deal of practice is likely to succeed in accomplishing.

Salt water spoils a looking-glass, and it would

therefore be necessary to wrap it up well out of harm's way; and, if it were greased thoroughly over its back and edges, it could be carried with still less risk. Finally, the mirror could only be used in moderate and sunshiny weather, but, with these restrictions, I believe it to afford a most valuable signal.

Obediently yours,

FRANCIS GALTON.

April 24.

Appendix C

Meteor.

TO THE EDITOR OF THE TIMES.[1]

Sir,—I was at Boulogne this morning at 11 o'clock, when a violent explosion followed by a low and long-continued rumbling, was heard in the Hotel des Bains, where I was then staying. The people in the house ran in alarm from their rooms into the courtyard asking one another what had happened. Then observing through the gateway that similar crowds were also collecting in the street and by the harbour and were equally puzzled as to the source of the noise, I went out, and found myself in ample time to see the long, narrow, smoke-like train of a meteor hanging in the sky. The final puff that indicated the place of explosion was marked with perfect distinctness, but the point where the train first commenced was hidden

[1] Galton 1866.

from my view by a block of houses. I leisurely remarked the necessary bearings and then running back to my room returned with a small travelling "altazimuth" I had by me, and measured them. The results were for the first point in the train that I could see, altitude, 62 deg.; magnetic azimuth, 95 deg; for the final puff, altitude, 40 deg.; magnetic azimuth, 195 deg.

I doubt the error in any of these observations exceeding 1 deg.; I feel sure it does not exceed 2 deg. The average breadth of the train of smoke was about 1 deg. A comparison of these measurements with any set taken elsewhere—and doubtless you will receive some other communication—will at least indicate the path of the meteor, and will accurately fix its height above the earth at the time of explosion.

FRANCIS GALTON.

Appendix D

Telegraphing to Mars.

MR. FRANCIS GALTON, in the *Times* of this day week, proposes seriously that our astronomers should agree on an attempt to flash sun-signals to Mars for several consecutive years, in the hope that they might attract attention from the possible inhabitants of Mars, and get us signals back of the same kind.[1] Whether the proposal to send such solar signals to Mars is possible or not can hardly be determined until we have some reason to presume that creatures like ourselves, in something like the same stage of knowledge as ourselves, exist on Mars, and that, we fear, is just what it is quite impossible to conjecture with any confidence sufficiently strong to inspire even a faint hope of success. If there be any truth in the assumption that on the amount of solar heat received

[1] Spectator, August 13, 1892, 218–219. See also Galton 1892.

at the surface of a planet depends the rate of progress in civilisation, it would be reasonable to suppose that even if such creatures as men exist on the planet Mars, they are not improbably behind us in the stage of their civilisation, and that telescopes may be as unknown to them as they were to our forefathers three or four thousand years ago; while if we assume an analogy of that kind to be illegitimate, then it must be still less legitimate to suppose that there is any analogy at all between our condition and theirs, even if they exist. The Martials, if there be Martials in any sense in which there are terrestrials on our own planet, may have no eyes at all; their whole civilisation, if they have any, may depend on senses of which we have absolutely no trace, so that communication between us and them would be a great deal less possible than communication between a fish and a mole, or between a blind man and a deaf mute. The whole idea of communicating with the inhabitants of Mars takes for granted that the Martials are organised more or less like ourselves, and especially in relation to the sense which carries farthest,—that is, the sense of sight. It would be an idle thing to send mere signals for consecutive years to a planet on which, even if there were rational beings, there was no sense of sight; and not very rational if, even though there were a sense of sight akin to our own, there was no power of aiding it by the help of telescopic inventions. Therefore it seems to us that unless the whole conception of communicating with Mars be in the highest degree extravagant, we have some reason to assume that the possible Martials are behind, not before us, in their stage of development and civilisation. We know that the tribes upon our earth which live under the most unfavourable conditions as regards heat,—the Esquimaux, for instance, and the Patagonians,—are far behind the inhabitants of the temperate regions in civilisation, and therefore, if we may draw any inferences at all as to the Martials from our own condition, the more probable inference is that, if they exist under circumstances at all like our own, they are, considering their great distance from the sun, centuries behind us rather than at the same stage of evolution, or still less centuries before us. And if we have no right to draw such an inference, then we have still less to reason with the smallest confidence from our own circumstances to theirs. They may, of course, have senses such as we have not even a dream of; they may be perfectly well acquainted with all that happens not only on our globe, but on all the other planets, and yet quite unable to let us know that they are familiar with our conditions of life, and how they have acquired that knowledge. But if that were so, it would be only too obvious that our conditions of life furnish us with no basis for forming any conjecture at all as to theirs; and in that case it would not only be sanguine, but quite irrational, to attempt to open communications at all. The only shadow of justification for making such an attempt rests on the assumption that we may reason from the. analogy of our own condition to theirs; and on that assumption we think it would be only prudent to assume that if such faculties as ours are already developed on the surface of Mars at all, they are likely to be far behind instead of far before our own.

But there is a further question of still more importance in connection with Mr. Galton's proposal. Let it be granted, for the sake of argument, that the Martials have eyes like ours and telescopes like ours, and that we could make them see our sun-flashes, and at last respond to them—how are we to establish any sort of code of communication without being able to establish any sort of association between our sun-flashes and the ideas we want to express?

Suppose, for example, that we wish to inquire the meaning and character of the long, straight canals on Mars, which have seemed to some of our observers artificial waterways of some kind, if they are not a vast deal too wide to be canals at all, or to ask the origin of those bright protuberances which some of our observers fancy to be artificial lights kindled on purpose to attract the attention of eyes in the nearest of Mars's planetary neighbours, how are we to set about asking the question, after we have satisfied ourselves, if we ever can satisfy ourselves, that the Martials see our signals and send us signals in return? When a human being finds himself amongst other human beings of whose language he is profoundly ignorant, he establishes at once some kind of association between sounds and wants, by the free use of signs. He points to his mouth, and makes the movements which accompany eating to express that he is hungry; or the movements which accompany drinking to express that he is thirsty; or he holds up his hands to signify entreaty and supplication; or he points to the East or West to indicate the direction from which he came; and he carefully attends to all the sounds which his hosts make, and so manages to associate one sound with food, another with drink, a third with the threatening or pleased expression of the strangers in whose power he finds himself, and a fourth with the word used for the quarter of space from which he has indicated that he had himself come. In that way, a code of intercourse is soon established, upon which some sort of mutual understanding is gradually built up. But how is any such code to be established with people whom we can neither see nor hear, nor make a Sign to of any kind, except the sign from which we infer that they are watching our sun-flashes as well as that we are watching theirs? Suppose we find that three flashes of ours are answered after a short interval by three flashes of theirs, and that ten flashes of ours are answered after the same interval by ten of theirs, we may then fairly assume that they understand us when we say three or ten, and that they have the faculty of number in common with us. But how are we to get any further? How are we to express a question of any sort, or to indicate the shape of the Martial canals and convey our curiosity, or to ask whether the bright prominences in Mars are artificial lights or glaciers at the tops of mountains catching the sunlight? We do not see how, if Mr. Galton had successfully made his first step, he could get any further, unless he could find the means of magnifying indefinitely, and then illuminating intensely, the face of a human being, so as to render it visible in Mars, with some sort of gesture or expression with which definite sun-signals could be associated. And as that of course is,—at present, at all events,—far beyond the range of scientific possibility, it seems to us that even the first step could not be made in arranging any kind of communication beyond that which assures us that number is common to us and to them. Suppose we telegraph two, and then three, and then are answered by five flashes from Mars, that might go to show that two and three make five in Mars as well as in the earth,—which Mr. J. S. Mill was, we suppose, slightly inclined to doubt, though that appears to us a doubt of the most irrational kind, which might justify a much deeper doubt, namely, whether the Martials had any capacity for either doubt or certainty. But after telegraphing any number of addition sums, and finding them properly answered from Mars, how are we to get as far as applying the conception of number to any concrete thing? How are we to ask if Martials have engineers and ships, and electric lights and glaciers, and five senses, and heads and feet, or to convey that we have them, unless we can contrive to send at least some few pictures to Mars and to get a pictorial reply, which is, we take it, at present beyond hope. We do not believe that astronomers will be content to go on flashing sun-signals for years to come to hypothetical Martial observers, only on the chance that. after the lapse of years or centuries, we may have the satisfaction of ascertaining that the faculty of number exists as much in Mars as it does in the earth, and that addition-sums are the same there that they are here, which seems to us already certain, if they have intelligences at all. It is, of course, barely possible that we may be able to discover for ourselves the nature of the so-called canals, which must be hundreds of miles in width, and whether the bright points are points of natural or artificial illumination; and if that could be discovered, we might then gradually learn more; but until we can clearly discover the form and character of some one Martial structure, living or otherwise, and convey to Mars the impression of some one real object here, we confess that there seems to us very little use in flashing sun-signals on the bare chance of proving that elementary arithmetic is understood in Mars as well as here.

Appendix E

Additional Notes

E.1 Philosophy

Clear mind from cant[1]

What G signifies to different persons

Infinitude is something larger than the largest conceivable — but what is that to different persons?

Take characters from good fiction

Ideals may well be elusive

The [imaginary] [case] Saints, VM, X,[2] [unites]

---

[1] p. f.1r.

[2] Virgin Mary, Christ.

[Agm[3]] Mahdi Mind
Honour Loyalty
[Animals witchery] relieves —bird [plovers] ants

Discipline (shipwreck) glory ambition emulation love hate family

E.2 Classification and Discontinuity

Trustworthiness of classification[4] applied to continuous variables

Small retail—Orange, Egg

Classes in Exam?

Passing recruits

Sentences

Cab fares—busses

Bribery

---

[3] Possibly 'annual general meeting', as in collective mind.
[4] p. f1.v.

Estimates of value of property

Doses of medicine

Salaries

E.3 Discontinuity

See Distinction between Compounds & Mixtures by P. J. Hartog[5] with reference to organic stability[6]

Possibilities of forms of [Chemicals]
see address

Geometric forms of simple organisms

classif: &c. [tastes] in
Nat. Sel. the same percentage die in each gen^{n} in a [static] pop. Those who survive stand an equal chance of continuity [of] their breed

Shrub & tree On the liability to E[rror] in arb[itary] Cla[ssification] [YMCV]
[Math.] ~~Error contingent on an arbitrary classif. of a~~

[5] P. J. Hartog 'On the Distinction between Mixtures and Compounds', read before the British Association, 1894.
[6] p. f4.

~~continuous variable~~

E.4 Botanical Notes on Heritability.

F. A. Dixey MD Wadham College Oxford April 9 / 95[7]

Entom: Soc: Trans 1887 pp 310–312

" " Proc: 1887 pp xvii xviii

Transmission of pink tubercles in Saturnia Carpini[8]

F. Merrifield 24 Vernon Terrace Brighton April 7 / 95

[Selenia Illustraria] 4 of a dark bronze colour that breed true[9]

Rev. G. Henslow Charminster Vicarage Dorchester (? permanent address)

April 12 / 95

Parsnips. The French long ago raised varieties, but

---

7 p. f7.

8 Emperor Moth.

9 'I thought that some data which were needed might be obtained by breeding insects, without too great expenditure of time and money, and it ended in my selecting for the purpose, under the advice of Mr. Merrifield, a particular kind of Moth, the "Selenia illustraria," which breeds twice a year and is hardy', Galton 1908, 307.

Prof Buckman sowing seed of the wild parsnips, raised similar varieties Radishes long a short-rooted.[10] Mr. Carriere[11] sowing seeds of the wild radish raised them by growing them in a loose & in a heavy soil an old fact recorded by Pliny & lately corroborated by the carrot. These varieties became fixed by selection & are quite hereditary by seed.

Parsnip Prof: Buckman neglecting all varieties but one fixed it in 1850 & called it the "student".[12] It is still the best in the trade. Spinescence due to drought—in wet climates the spines are lost Characters have every degree of persistence Question suggested "Are the varieties or specific characters constant under a changed environment? If not, to what extent are they hereditary, or how do they alter?" The wild cabbage, and the wild sea kale, have no varieties when under natural conditions.

I do not understand the following — "Many garden plants show innumerable variations as either two species of the same genus are not in cultivation as the sweet pea, cabbage, Pansy, cineraria; or else the species will not cross with others as the many 'races' which have

[10] variety

[11] E. A. Carrière.

[12] James Buckman (1814–1884) was at the Royal Agriculture College in Cirencester, England.

been established by selection among seedlings of the Chinese primrose."

Instances given of effects of environment—all Alpine plants tend to be dwarf ... desert to be spinescent; acquatic to have finely [...] or ribbon-like submerged leaves.

His pamphlet is enclosed on "The Origin of Species without the aid of Natural Selection" reprinted from "Natural Science" vol. V No 32 Oct 1894. It is a reply to an article by A. R. Wallace No. 31, Sept 1894.

E.5 Botanical Notes on Heritability (2).

Haycraft Darwinism &c. Swan & Sonnenschein / 95[13][14]
p 40 Among plants it really appears as if by adjusting the soil & the climate you may produce stunted varieties whose seed produce small plants. A classical case mentioned by Lemaire (D'Orbigny's dictio-

[13] John Berry Haycraft (1859–1922) *Darwinism and Race Progress* (London: Swan and Sonnenschein, 1895).
[14] p. f8r.

nary[15]) is that of the [Hera] when removed from Piedmont to France become a smaller variety only ½ its former height, in 2 or 3 generations

Pointing, begging & retrieving of dogs.
sheep tending.

Mrs. McLennan geraniums

Baron v. Maltzan on the People of South Arabia, read before the Berlin Anthropological Society in 1873 or / 72 He "refers to the existence among the Himyarites of families in which the possession of six fingers on the hand is hereditary. The sixth finger is considered by the people a sign of blue blood. The observations ... are deserving of translation, but we have not space." Anthropologica I Oct 1873 (first publication of the London Anthropological Society founded Jan / 73)[16]

Revd F. Bennett
Farley Rectory Warlingham Surrey 50

[15] Charles D'Orbigny (1802-1857) *Dictionnaire Universel d'Histoire Naturelle* (1849).
[16] *Anthropologica* Vol. I, October 1873, p. 115.

E.6 Botanical Notes on Heritability (3).

Hubert Airy Proc. R. Soc[17]
(1) Feb 27 / 1873 p 176 Leaf arrangement
(2) March 23 / 1874 p. 298 " "
(3) May 8 / 1876 p 158 Cranberry

Shows that the *maxima* of stability are at the terms of the $\frac{1}{3}, \frac{2}{5}, \frac{3}{8}, \frac{5}{13}$ &c. [series] The particular term depending on the distance of the ball from the India rubber band

A variability per saltum in no. of vertical [ranks] is a reasonable hypothesis 1874 p 304

"... it does not seem possible that one could be produced from another by accumulative 'modification' see Summary p 307

Compare however with 1876 p 160 where one series in the cranberry is frequently turned into another by unequal condensation resulting in spiral dislocation

17 p. f10.

E.7 Fingerprint Data.

[Editor: Brief fingerprint data for Dorothy and Muriel Brooke][18]

E.8 Botanical Notes on Heritability (4).

J Buckman Report in Experimental plots at the Agricult: coll: Cirencester Journ Brit: Assocn 200[19]
p. 202 Agrostis—the three forms Agr. vulgaris, alba & stolonifera seem referable to a simple species.[20] The seed of one, though for the most part coming true will still send up exceptional examples of each of the others. A. vulgaris is common in upland meadows, A. alba in ditches & damp places. A stolonifera in strong bushes &c.

Festuca loliacea, pratensis, and elatior[21] are similarly shown by experiment to be all referable to a single species. (1) grows true in meadows by the sides of rivers (2) in rich meadow flats. (3) on alluvial sandy clay banks by the seaside or poor siliceous clays instead Journ. Brit Assoc 1860 p. 35 These experi-

[18] p. f11.
[19] p. f16b.
[20] Bent grass.
[21] Meadow grass.

ments with Festuca repeated successfully

p. 39 Pastinaca Sativa Parsnip—the Student Parsnip (only alluded to)[22] Brassica Oleracea, Wild Cabbage. Its seeds produced plants showing tendency to run into many of the cabbage varieties long petioles—Kale, greens, &c. both with broad, more or less undivided leaves, and with a tendency to deep lobes and divisions.

The paper in 1859 does not help me

E.9 Balfour's Foundations of Belief.

Foundations of belief. A. J. Balfour[23]
Longmans 1895.[24]

5. Kant requires to be rethought by Enlightenment & reproduced in a form the Englishmen will assimilate. Chap I Naturalising Ethics

11. The substance of the moral law is accepted by

[22] Wild parsnip.
[23] p. f57a.
[24] Arthur James Balfour (1848–1930) was Prime Minister, 1902–1905. *The foundations of belief; being notes introductory to the study of theology, by the Right Hon. Arthur James Balfour* went through many editions. Balfour contested the idea that Darwinism undermined religion.

all but the grounds on which they accept it differ. (? as to this—Code of honour & duelling in a Xtn[25] society—war Effort of western nations as against quietude — celibacy/ Claims of family & of state ...)

13. No moral code can be effective which does not inspire reverence (1) (? reverence is a compound of love & fear. A moral code may be based on either separately. Love—The children carrying out the mere fancies of a deceased parent; loyalty, self-sacrifice of a lover Mother's teachings. Fear of the world's opinion, of the law of an autocrat. Discipline.)

13. The capacity of a code to excite reverence &c. cannot be wholly (2) independent of its accepted origin. (His estimate of naturalism seems to me a gross exaggeration of what necessarily follows from his description of it p. 7 Emotional capacity, aesthetic &c. must potentially exist in the material out of which we are made. They may be almost infinitesimal in each particle but the battery of a vast multitude of organised particles gives finite effects.)

14 &c. He concludes from (2) that the naturalistic creed cannot excite reverence.

[25] Christian.

18 Kant composes the moral law to the starry heavens. The naturalist might compose it to the protective blotches on a beetle's back.[26]

Determinism & free will. He suggests p. 20 that the dilution of free will must on the naturalistic hypothesis be the result of natural selection, the fatalists in practice perishing.

21. The comedy of all mankind except a few believing themselves free while the latter act as if they were so.

22 Savages certainly believe in their own freedom because they attribute spontaneity to natural objects, anthropomorphically. A foot note throws doubt on the absolute uniformity of Nature—"at the moment of choice no uniformity of antecedents need ensure a uniformity of consequences" (the inveterate illusion)

24 A fatalistic tendency is found in the minds of some of the greatest men of action, which does not weaken their volition but

[26] 'Kant, as we all know, compared the Moral Law to the starry heavens, and found them both sublime. It would, on the naturalistic hypothesis, be more appropriate to compare it to the protective blotches on the beetle's back, and to find them both ingenious'.

E.10 Balfour's Foundations of Belief (continued).

adds a finer temper to their courage. Still in general belief in determinism does really conflict with the sense of personal responsibility.[27]

25 The admiration accorded to a virtuous man would become like that we now accord to a well made machine.

26 (1) Are the ends prescribed by morality adequate? (on the naturalistic hypothesis) conflict between egoism & altruism, unequal distribution of happiness with
27 no future state to set matters right.

28 Emotional adequacy—felicity of the sentient creation—but man's action
29 is so unimportant, moreover he is (naturalistically) a mere accident (fine passage about the blunderings & vileness of man)

32 Our practical ideal is beggared by these thoughts

Chap II Naturalism & Aesthetic

[27] p. f57b.

33. Aesthetics useless for preservation must be by-products Take music as free from objections to the rest (architecture & utility &c. A preexisting taste is needed to cause the favourable variation.

38 Spencer's muscular [contraction] "of the abdomen &c. and the noises there deduced have association &c. absurdity of it. The sounds that 41 have associations give no delight & those that give delight have no assoc.

Discordant views of beauty—critical traditions.

The outfit of a critic is as much intellectual as emotional.
50 fashion in dress

The general tendency to agreement—sets & coteries

59 The arts progress but the pleasure given by them to each successive generation does not seem to increase.

Chap III Naturalism & Reason

67 The non-rational origin of reason (Is this fair?)

69 It is most improbable that our senses are even approximately adequate

73 Reason creates habits by wh: it is itself supplanted

75 Spencer's trust that man will become so perfectly adapted to his surroundings that goodness will be automatic—but so will reason & all that time we shall be idiotic. Sensibly poorer by this deposition of reason from its ancient position to that of an expedient for maintaining organic life.

Chap IV Summary of Part I[28]

E.11 Encoding.

[Editor: first page with numerical encoding in terms of dots and dashes][29]

E.12 Encoding Rhumbs and Decimals

Another trial Jul 29 / 96[30]
with 24 rhumbs and decimals.

[28] There are no more sections in the notebook on Balfour.
[29] p. f59.
[30] p. f67r.

E.

[...]

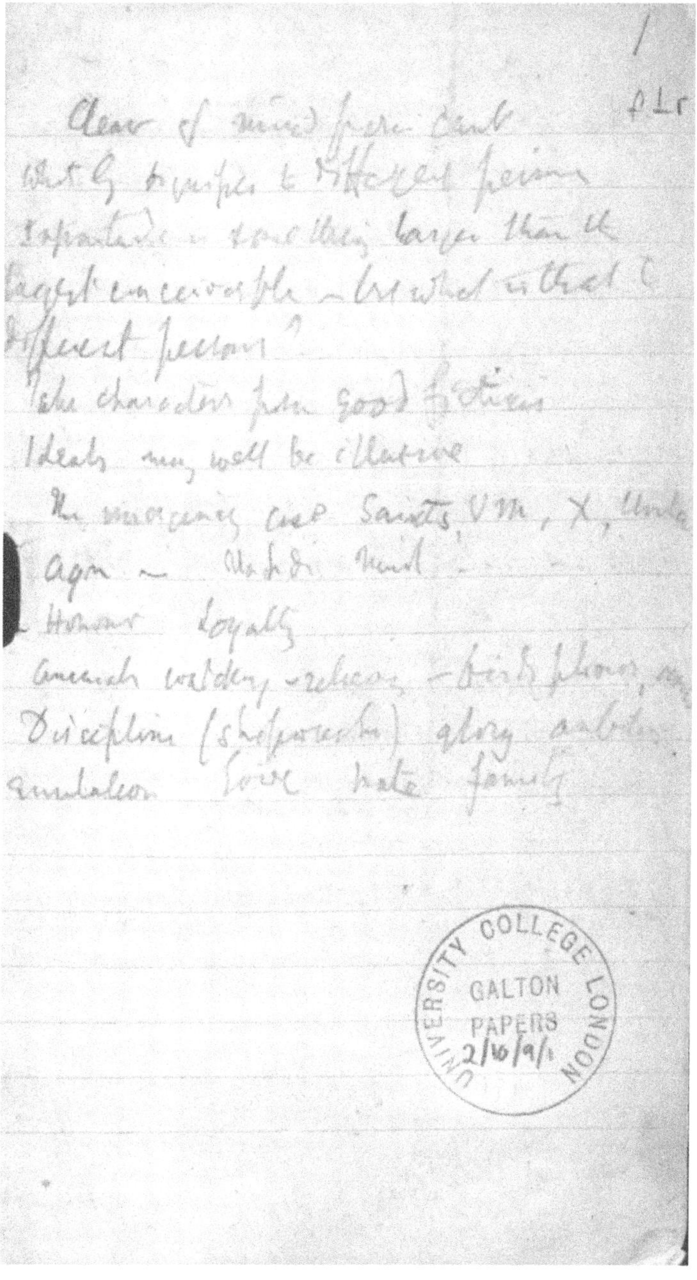

Figure E.1: Page f1r. Philosophy.

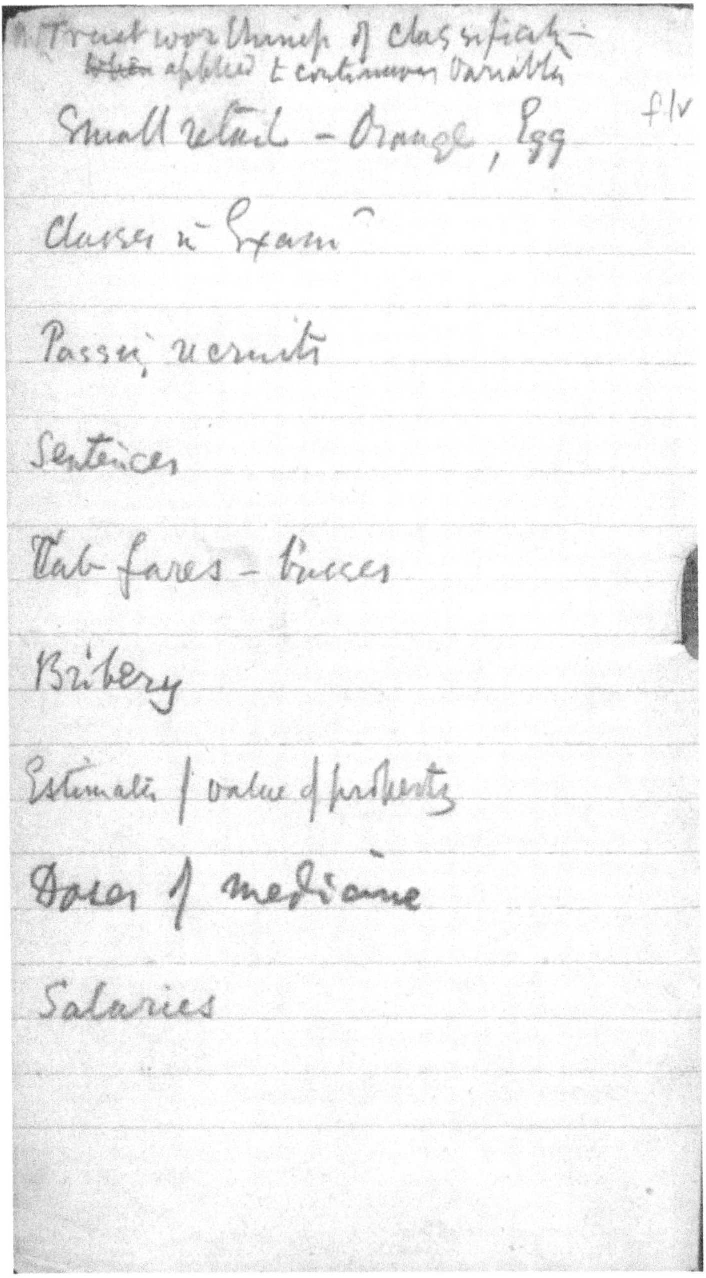
1. Trustworthiness of classification –
when applied to continuous variables
f1v
Small retail – Orange, Egg
Classes in Exam
Passing recruits
Sentences
Cab fares – buses
Bribery
Estimate of value of property
Doses of medicine
Salaries

Figure E.2: Page f1v. Discontinuity.

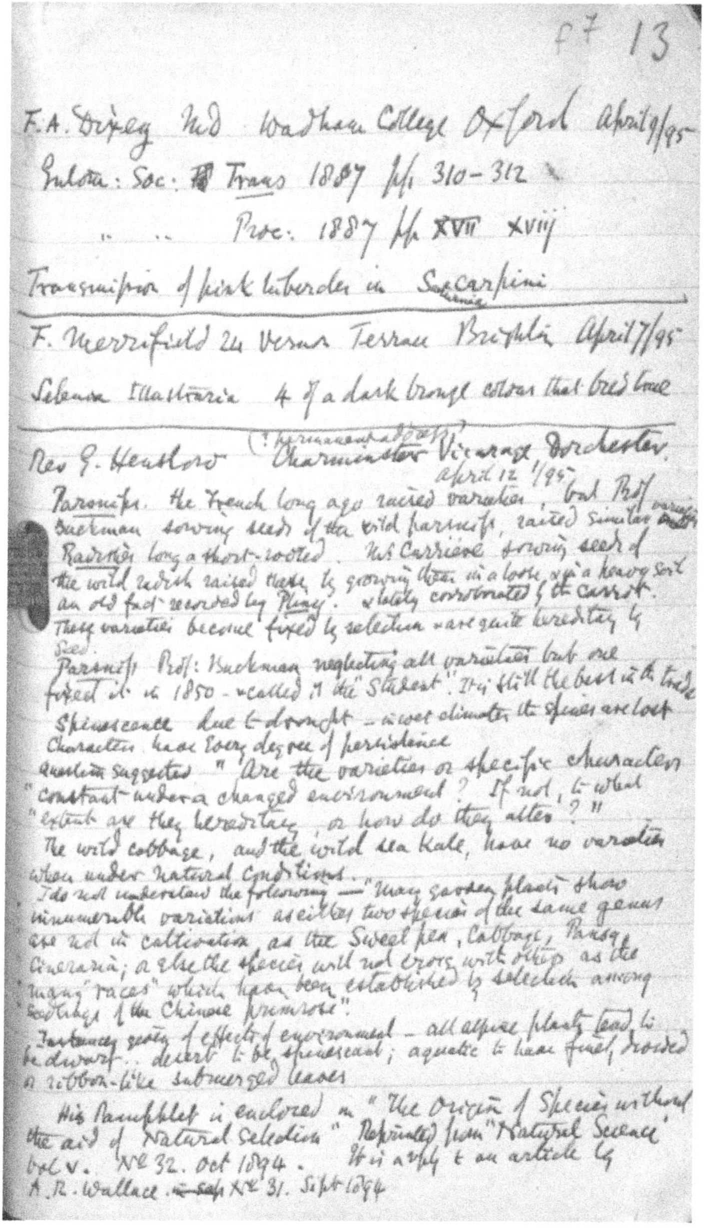
f7 13

F. A. Dixey M.D. Wadham College Oxford April 9/95
Entom: Soc: Trans 1887 pp. 310-312
" " Proc: 1887 pp XVII XVIII
Transmission of pink tubercles in Saccarpini
F. Merrifield 24 Vernon Terrace Brighton April 7/95
Selenia Illustraria 4 of a dark orange colour that bred true
Rev G. Henslow (? permanent address) Charminster Vicarage, Dorchester.
April 12 1/95
Parsnips. the French long ago raised varieties, but Prof Buckman sowing seeds of the wild parsnips, raised similar varieties
Radishes long & short-rooted. M. Carrière sowing seeds of the wild radish raised these by growing them in a loose, or in a heavy soil an old fact recorded by Pliny. & lately corroborated of the carrot.
These variations become fixed by selection & are quite hereditary by seed.
Parsnips Prof: Buckman neglecting all variations but one fixed it in 1850 - & called it the "Student". It is still the best in the trade
Spinescence due to drought - in wet climates the spines are lost
Characters have every degree of persistence
question suggested "Are the variations or specific characters "constant under a changed environment? If not, to what "extent are they hereditary, or how do they alter?"
The wild cabbage, and the wild sea kale, have no variation when under natural conditions.
I do not understand the following — "Many garden plants show "innumerable variations as either two species of the same genus "are not in cultivation, as the Sweet pea, Cabbage, Pansy, "Cineraria; or else the species will not cross with others as the "many "races" which have been established by selection among "seedlings of the Chinese primrose".
Instances given of effects of environment - all alpine plants tend to be dwarf... desert to be spinescent; aquatic to have finely divided or ribbon-like submerged leaves
His Pamphlet is enclosed in "The Origin of Species without the aid of Natural Selection" Reprinted from "Natural Science" Vol V. No 32. Oct 1894. It is a reply to an article by A. R. Wallace. No 31. Sept 1894

Figure E.3: Page f7. Heritability.

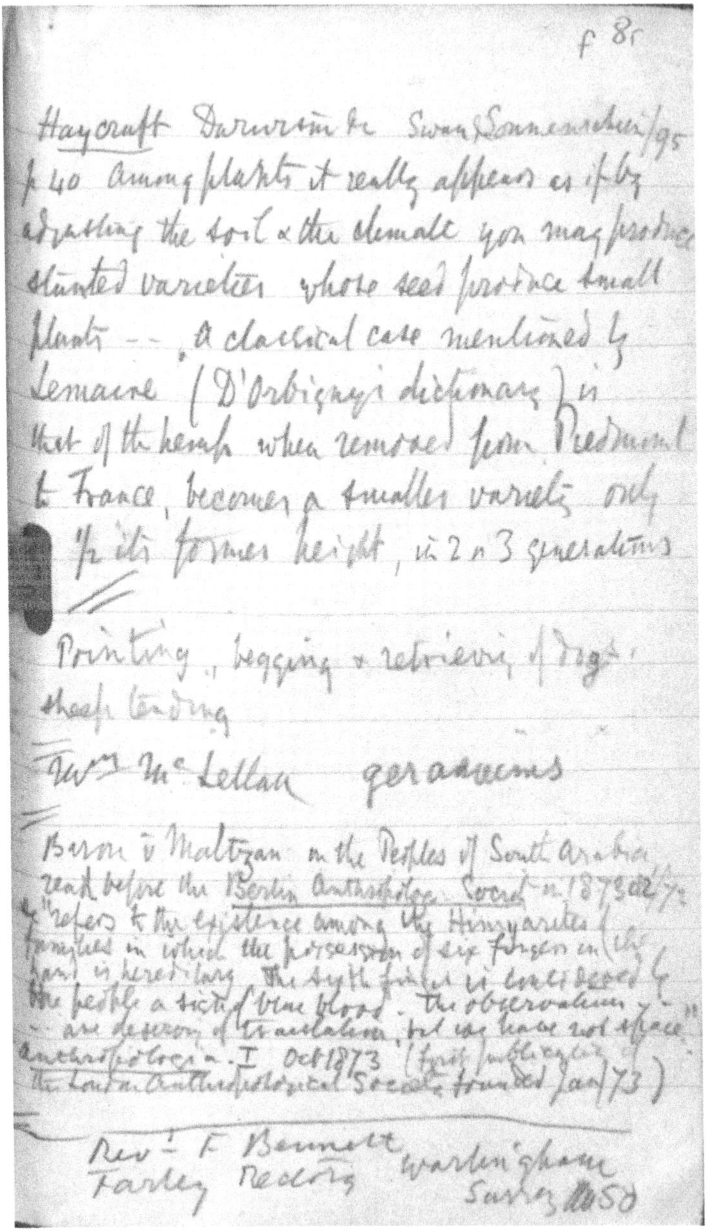

f 8r

Haycraft Darwinism &c Swan Sonnenschein/95
p 40 among plants it really appears as if by
adjusting the soil & the climate you may produce
stunted varieties whose seed produce small
plants -- "a classical case mentioned by
Lemaire (D'Orbigny's dictionary) is
that of the hemp when removed from Piedmont
to France, becomes a smaller variety only
1/2 its former height, in 2 or 3 generations

//

Pointing, begging & retrieving of dogs.
sheep tending

Wm McLellan geraniums

//

Baron v Maltzan on the Peoples of South Arabia
read before the Berlin Anthropolog. Society in 1873
"refers to the existence among the Himyarites of
families in which the possession of six fingers on the
hand is hereditary. The sixth finger is considered by
the people a sign of blue blood. The observations
-- are deserving of translation, but we have not space"
Anthropologia. I Oct 1873 (first publication of
The London Anthropological Society founded Jan/73)

Revd F Bennett Farley Rectory Warlingham Surrey

Figure E.4: Page f8r. Heritability.

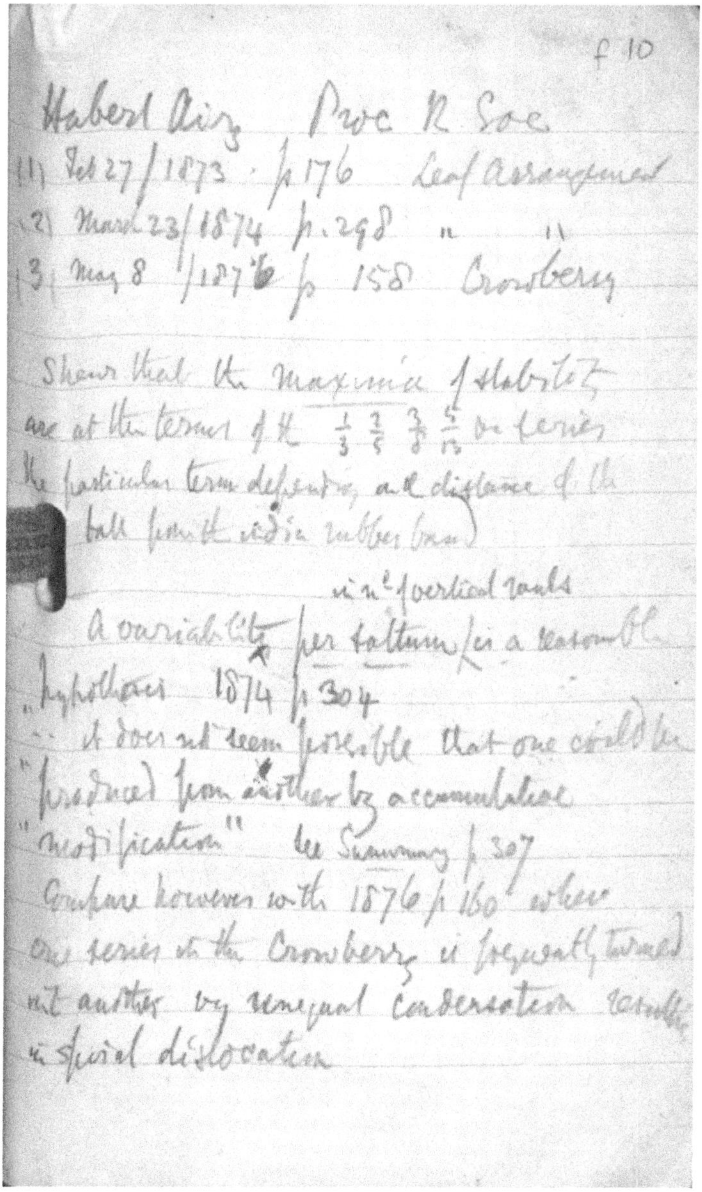

f 10

Hubert Airy Proc R Soc
(1) Feb 27/1873 . p 176 Leaf Arrangement
(2) March 23/1874 p. 298 " "
(3) May 8 /1876 p 158 Crowberry

Shows that the maxima of stability are at the terms of the $\frac{1}{3}$ $\frac{2}{5}$ $\frac{3}{8}$ $\frac{5}{13}$ &c series the particular term depending on distance of the balls from the india rubber band)

in n^e of vertical ranks
A variability per pattern for a reasonable hypothesis 1874 p 304
"it does not seem possible that one could be "produced from another by accumulative "modification" see Summary p 307
Compare however with 1876 p 160 where one series in the Crowberry is frequently turned into another by unequal condensation resulting in spiral dislocation

Figure E.5: Page f10. Heritability.

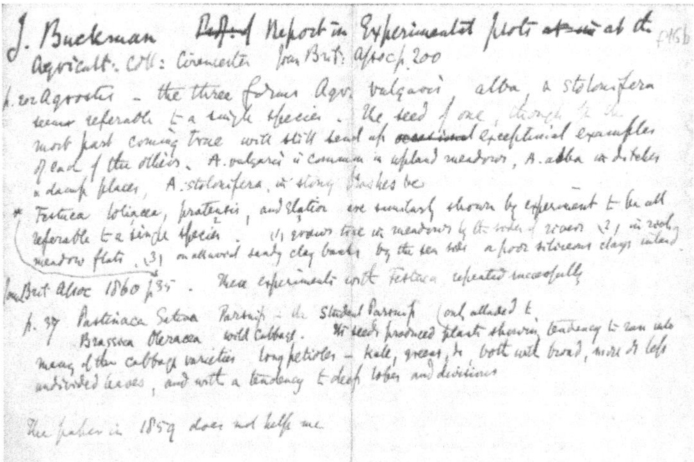
J. Buckman ~~Rep~~ Report on Experimental plots ~~at~~ at the f16b
Agricult. Coll: Cirencester Jour Brit. Assoc p. 200
p. 202 Agrostis – the three forms Agr. vulgaris, alba, & stolonifera
seem referable to a single species. The seed of one, though for the
most part coming true will still send up ~~occasional~~ exceptional examples
of each of the others. A. vulgaris is common in upland meadows, A. alba in ditches
& damp places, A. stolonifera in stony banks &c
* Festuca loliacea, pratensis, and elatior are similarly shown by experiment to be all
referable to a single species. (1) grows true in meadows by the sides of rivers (2) in rocky
meadow flats, (3) on alluvial sandy clay banks by the sea side & poor siliceous clays inland
Jour Brit Assoc 1860 p 35. These experiments with Festuca repeated successfully
p. 37 Pastinaca Sativa Parsnip – the Student Parsnip (only alluded to
Brassica Oleracea wild Cabbage. The seeds produced plants showing tendency to run into
many of the cabbage varieties long petioles – kale, greens, &c both with broad, more or less
undivided leaves, and with a tendency to deep lobes and divisions
The paper in 1859 does not help me

Figure E.6: Page f16b. Heritability.

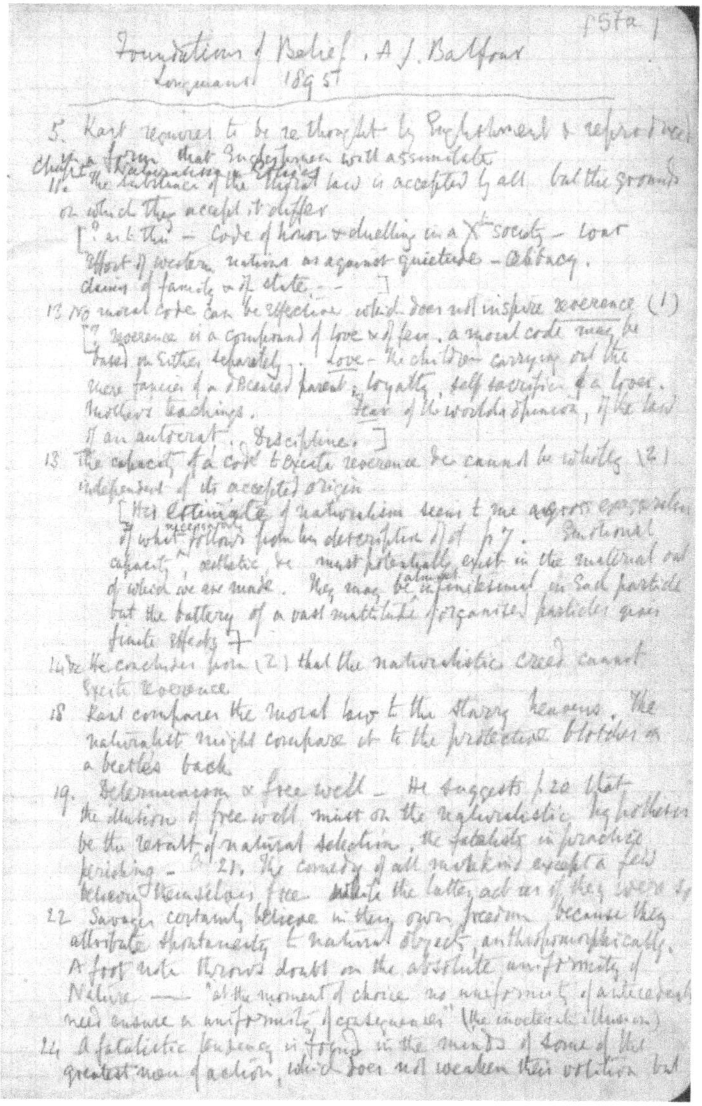

f57a 1

Foundations of Belief. A J. Balfour
Longmans 1895

5. Kant requires to be re thought by Englishmen & reformed [illegible] in a form that Englishmen will assimilate.
Chapt. 1 Naturalism & Ethics
11. The substance of the moral law is accepted by all but the grounds on which they accept it differ
[? as to this – Code of honor & duelling in a X^t society – love [illegible] of western nations as against quietude – celibacy. claims of family & of state. – –]
13 No moral code can be effective which does not inspire reverence (1)
[? reverence is a compound of love & of fear. a moral code may be based on either separately. Love – the children carrying out the mere fancies of a deceased parent, loyalty, self sacrifice of a lover. Mother's teachings. Fear of the world's opinion, of the law of an autocrat, Discipline.]
13. The capacity of a code to excite reverence &c cannot be wholly (2) independent of its accepted origin
[His estimate of naturalism seems to me a gross exaggeration of what necessarily follows from his description of it p 7. Emotional capacity, aesthetic &c must potentially exist in the material out of which we are made. They may be (almost) infinitesimal in each particle but the battery of a vast multitude of organized particles gives finite effects]
14 He concludes from (2) that the naturalistic creed cannot excite reverence
18 Kant compares the moral law to the starry heavens. The naturalist might compare it to the protective blotches on a beetle's back
19. Determinism & free will – He suggests p 20 that the illusion of free will must on the naturalistic hypothesis be the result of natural selection, the fatalists in practice perishing – 21. The comedy of all mankind except a few believing themselves free while the latter act as if they were so
22 Savages certainly believe in their own freedom because they attribute spontaneity to natural objects, anthropomorphically. A foot note throws doubt on the absolute uniformity of Nature — "at the moment of choice no uniformity of antecedents need ensure a uniformity of consequences" (the [illegible] illusion)
24 A fatalistic tendency is found in the minds of some of the greatest men of action, which does not weaken their volition but

Figure E.7: Page f57a. Balfour.

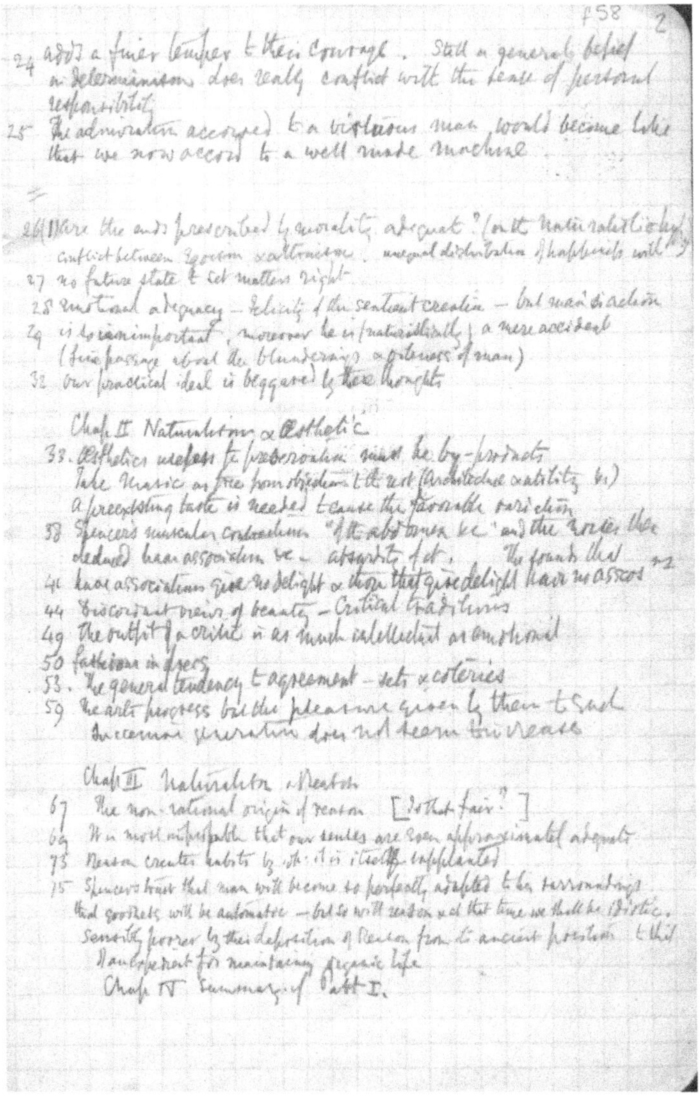

f58 2

24 adds a finer temper to their courage. Still a general belief in Determinism does really conflict with the sense of personal responsibility

25 The admiration accorded to a virtuous man would become like that we now accord to a well made machine.

26 (Were the ends prescribed by morality adequate? (on the naturalistic hyp.) conflict between Egoism & altruism. unequal distribution of happiness with

27 no future state to set matters right

28 emotional adequacy – felicity of the sentient creation – but man the actor

29 is too unimportant, moreover he is (naturalistically) a mere accident (fine passage about the blunderings & greatness of man)

32 Our practical ideal is beggared by these thoughts

Chap II Naturalism & Æsthetic

33. Æsthetics useless for preservation must be by-products
Take Music as free from objections to the rest (Architecture & utility &c)
A preexisting taste is needed to cause the favorable variation

38 Spencer's muscular contractions "of the abdomen &c" and the [illegible] [illegible] deduced from association &c – absurdity of it. The fact that

41 have associations give no delight & those that give delight have no assocs. *2

44 Discordant views of beauty – Critical traditions

49 The outfit of a critic is as much intellectual as emotional

50 fashions in dress

53. The general tendency to agreement – sets & coteries

59 The arts progress but the pleasure given by them to each successive generation does not seem to increase

Chap III Naturalism & Reason

67 The non-rational origin of reason [Is that fair?]

69 It is most [illegible] that our senses are even approximately adequate

73 Reason creates habits by which it is itself supplanted

75 Spencer's trust that man will become so perfectly adapted to his surroundings that[illegible] will be automatic – but so will reason & at that time we shall be idiotic. Sensibly [illegible] by this deposition of Reason from its ancient position to this [illegible] for maintaining organic life

Chap IV Summary of Part I.

Figure E.8: Page f57b. Balfour.

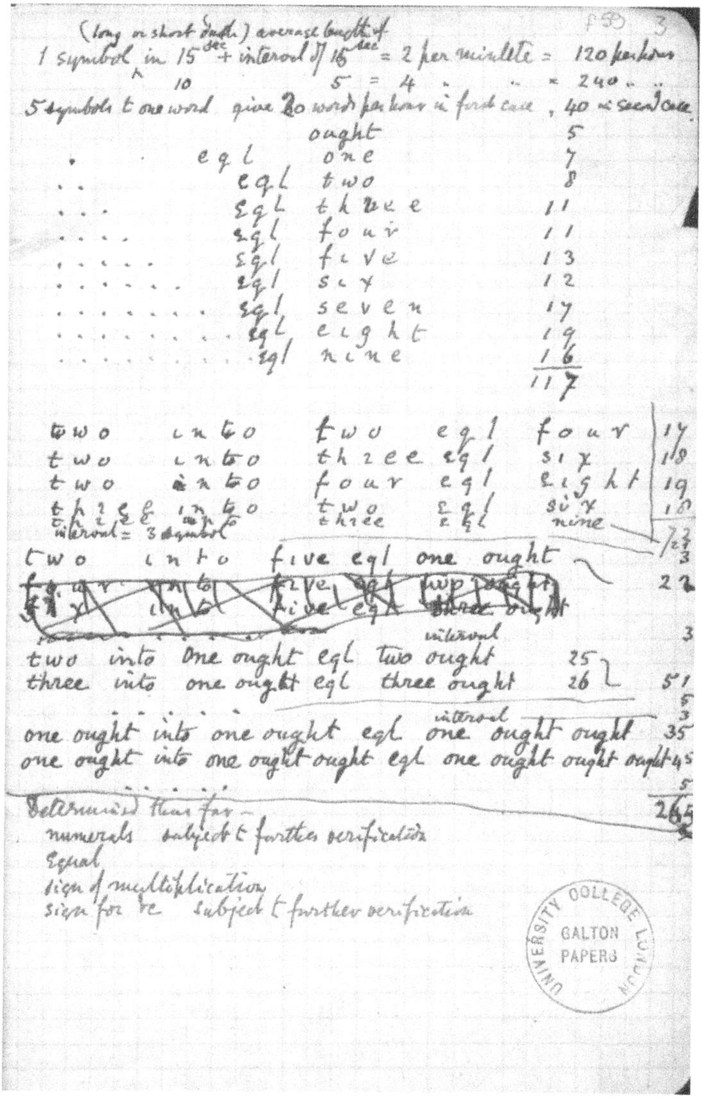

Figure E.9: Page f59. Encoding.

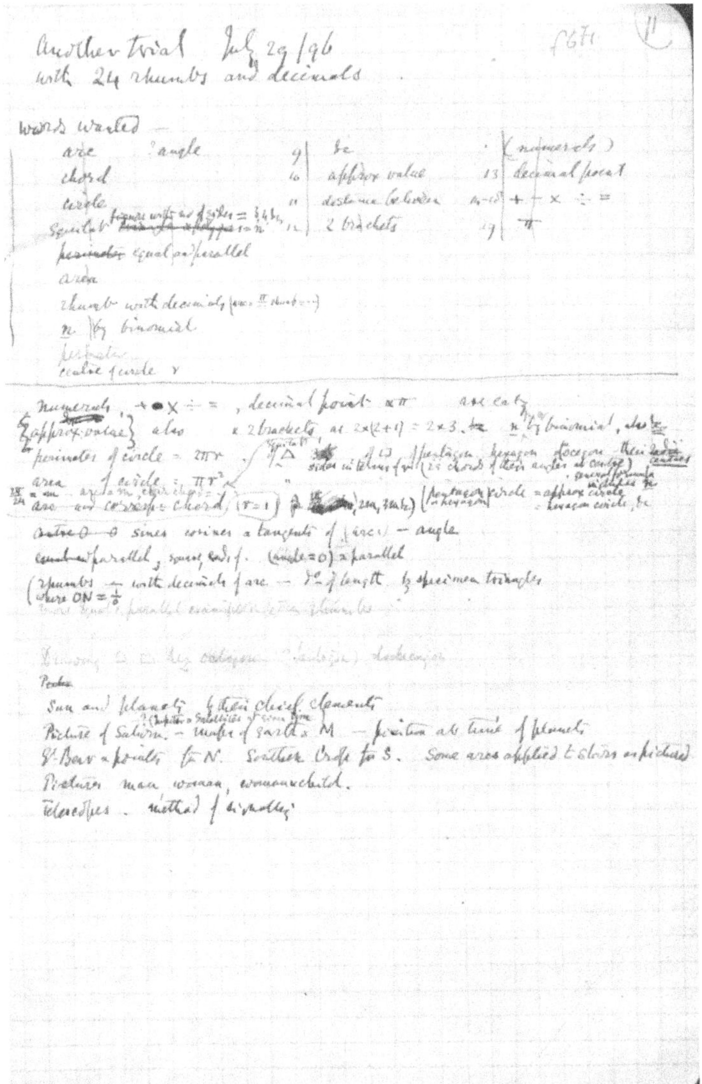

Figure E.10: Page f67r. Encoding.

List of Figures

Glossary

Chepmell, Dr. Isaac Dobrée

(1828–1919), educated at Elizabeth College and Kings College, and for at least 8 years the travelling personal physician of Lord Hollond. He was forced to retire in 1897, due to acute glaucoma. His other patients included Lady Gregory. See *Lancet*, Feb. 6, 1897, 394 17

Bibliography

Forrest, Derek William (1974). *Francis Galton. The Life and Work of a Victorian Genius*. London: Paul Elek, 1974.

Galton, Francis (1855). *The Art of Travel; or, Shifts and Contrivances Available in Wild Countries*. First edition. London: John Murray, 1855.

— (1856a). "Signals Available to Men who are Adrift on Wrecks at Sea." In: *Times* (Apr. 4, 1856), 10e.

— (1856b). *The Art of Travel; or, Shifts and Contrivances Available in Wild Countries*. Second edition. London: John Murray, 1856.

— (1858). "A description of a hand heliostat." In: *Report of the British Association for the Advancement of Science* (1858), pp. 211–212.

— (1860). *The Art of Travel; or, Shifts and Contrivances Available in Wild Countries*. Third edition. London: John Murray, 1860.

Galton, Francis, ed. (1861). *Vacation tourists and Notes of Travel in 1860*. London: Macmillan, 1861.

— (1866). "Meteor." In: *Times* (June 21, 1866), 7f.

— (1867). *The Art of Travel; or, Shifts and Contrivances Available in Wild Countries.* Fourth edition. London: John Murray, 1867.

— (1872). *The Art of Travel; or, Shifts and Contrivances Available in Wild Countries.* Fifth edition. London: John Murray, 1872.

— (1879). "Observations on the eclipse of 1860." In: *Memoirs of the Royal Astronomical Society* XLI (1879), pp. 563–564.

— (1892). "Sun Signals to Mars." In: *Times* (Aug. 6, 1892), 7f.

— (1893). "The just-perceptible difference." In: *Proceedings of the Royal Institution* 14 (Jan. 27, 1893), pp. 13–26.

— (1896a). "Intelligible signals between neighbouring stars." In: *Fortnightly Review* 60 (Nov. 1, 1896), pp. 657–64.

— (1896b). "Signalling from Mars." In: *London Evening Standard* (Oct. 29, 1896), p. 2.

— (1908). *Memories of My Life*. London: Methuen, 1908.

Tredoux, Gavan (2023). *Sir Francis Sacheverel Darwin*. galton.org, 2023.

Made in the USA
Monee, IL
04 November 2026

67387586R00095